J. GURNEY

Evidence-Based Diagnosis

Springer
New York
Berlin
Heidelberg
Barcelona
Hong Kong
London
Milan
Paris
Singapore
Tokyo

Mark H. Ebell, M.D., M.S.
Associate Professor
Department of Family Medicine
Michigan State University
CoDirector, Michigan Consortium for Family Practice Research

Evidence-Based Diagnosis: A Handbook of Clinical Prediction Rules

With 25 Illustrations

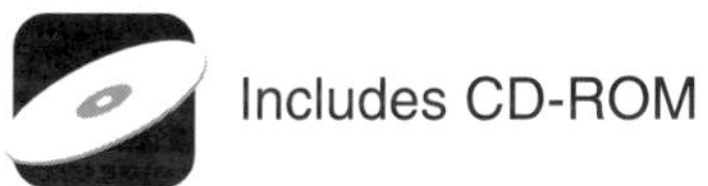
Includes CD-ROM

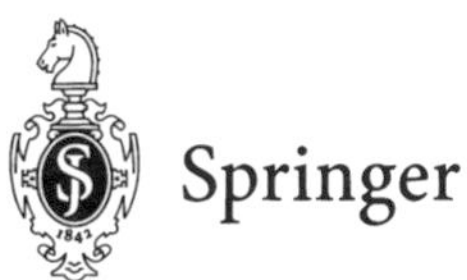
Springer

Mark H. Ebell, M.D., M.S.
Department of Family Medicine
Michigan State University
B101 Clinical Center
East Lansing, MI 48824
USA
ebell@pilot.msu.edu

Library of Congress Cataloging-in-Publication Data
Ebell, Mark H.
Evidence-based diagnosis : a handbook of clinical prediction rules / by Mark H. Ebell.
p. ; cm.
Includes bibliographical references and index.
ISBN 0-387-95025-7 (hard cover : alk. paper)
1. Diagnosis—Statistical methods—Handbooks, manuals, etc. 2. Evidence based medicine—Handbooks, manuals, etc. I. Title.
[DNLM: 1. Diagnosis—Handbooks. 2. Decision Support Techniques—Handbooks. 3. Evidence-Based Medicine—Handbooks. 4. Predictive Value of Tests—Handbooks. 5. Prospective Studies—Handbooks. WB 39 E15e 2000]
RC71.3 .E85 2000
616.07′5—dc21 00-026571

Printed on acid-free paper.

Production managed by MaryAnn Brickner; manufacturing supervised by Jacqui Ashri.
Typeset by Impressions Book and Journal Services, Inc., Madison, WI.
Printed and bound by Hamilton Printing Co., Rensselaer, NY.
Printed in the United States of America.

9 8 7 6 5 4 3 2 1

ISBN 0-387-95025-7 SPIN 10762955

Springer-Verlag New York Berlin Heidelberg
A member of BertelsmannSpringer Science+Business Media GmbH

This work is dedicated to my faithful writing companions:
Alex, Elvis, Kudzu, and Max.

Contents

1

Using Clinical Prediction Rules in Your Practice

How likely is a disease? What is a patient's prognosis? Can we expect surgery to be successful? Taking care of patients involves many predictions and estimates. Answering these questions accurately is critical for the physician who wants to provide high quality, cost-effective care for his or her patients. Traditionally, we have based these estimates and predictions on our judgment and clinical experience.

Unfortunately, clinical experience can be misleading. As humans we are "wired" to pay attention to the new, the unusual, and the interesting. We are not very good at making observations over time in a consistent, systematic, and unbiased way.

For one thing, personal experience with a few patients may be misleading; we all know that a single bad experience can inappropriately affect a clinician's practice pattern, even if that experience was a rare exception. Conversely, if a patient responds well to a new medication, we are much more likely to think that it will work for the next patient. Our experience in medical schools, often at tertiary care hospitals, may overexpose us to the rare and bizarre, with the result that we overestimate the likelihood of rare and bizarre outcomes.

The availability of information, as in a recent journal article, also heightens our awareness of a condition, and makes it more likely that we (rightly or wrongly) diagnose it in subsequent patients.[1] Finally, the opinions of colleagues and information in textbooks may be based on anecdotes rather than data about prevalence of disease and outcome. These and other biases limit our ability to make accurate diagnoses and prognoses for our patients.

How can we be more accurate? A *clinical prediction rule* (also called a decision rule or a predictive index) is a tool that takes the experience of a group of physicians with hundreds or even thousands of patients and distills this experience into a simple rule. By using the rule, we can make more accurate diagnoses and prognoses. Consider the following example.

> Your patient just underwent exercise electrocardiography to evaluate his chest pain. He had 1 mm of ST depression, exercised for 10 minutes, and the test was stopped owing to fatigue (the patient experienced no pain). How do you interpret this information? What is the likelihood he will suffer a cardiac event during the next 4 years? This question is important because if the likelihood of problems is high the patient should be evaluated more aggressively using cardiac catheterization; if it is low, he can be managed conservatively using medical management.

A clinical prediction rule has been developed to help physicians establish the prognosis of patients who have had an exercise electrocardiogram. Called the Treadmill Score, it assigns points to patients based on the type of chest pain experienced during the test (if any), the extent of ST segment depression (if any), and the duration of exercise.[2] Low scores are associated with a worse outcome. Thus a primary care physician can use the score to manage patients more effectively, reserving a more aggressive workup for those more likely to suffer a cardiac event during the next 4 years. For example, the above patient has a 99% four-year survival rate, so aggressive evaluation is probably not warranted.

Hundreds of clinical prediction rules have been developed, and many have been well validated. Well known examples include the Ottawa Ankle Rules, the Strep Score, the CAGE score for alcoholism, and the Treadmill Score described above. Unfortunately, it may be difficult to find clinical prediction rules in the literature, as there is no consistent way they are indexed. Once found, it is difficult to have them at hand when you need them. Many also require fairly complex calculations and are difficult to memorize. Perhaps most importantly, it is not often clear whether a rule has been tested thoroughly enough for the results to be believable. That is where this handbook comes in.

This book is the first of its kind: a collection of clinical prediction rules for use by clinicians. Each clinical prediction rule has been systematically evaluated, which helps you decide whether the rule should apply to your patients. Most of the clinical rules in this book have been validated in a separate group of patients to help ensure the rule's accuracy. Best of all, some of the best validated and most important rules have been translated into software for your desktop computer. I hope this book helps you become a "more rational" physician and in the process helps you and your patients make more informed decisions about their health care.

CLINICAL PREDICTION RULES AND EVIDENCE-BASED MEDICINE

Evidence-based medicine is an important new paradigm for the practice of medicine. Put simply, an evidence-based approach means that a physician should use the best available evidence when making a decision to use a diagnostic test or choose a treatment. Clinical prediction rules are a convenient and rapid way to apply the results of research to the care of patients and to help physicians make more accurate decisions.

For example, consider an ambulatory patient with a sore throat. One approach advocated by practitioners of evidence-based medicine is to prescribe penicillin if the likelihood of streptococcal pharyngitis is high, base the treatment decision on a rapid antigen screen if the likelihood is intermediate, and consider symptomatic treatment only if the likelihood of a streptococcal infection is low. Unfortunately, single elements of the history and physical examination are not good at predicting that likelihood. The Strep Score is a clinical prediction rule that combines four common clinical variables and accurately estimates the likelihood of streptococcal pharyngitis. To use it, count the number of the following clinical characteristics that are present: (1) history of fever; (2) anterior cervical adenopathy; (3) tonsilar exudate; and (4) absence of cough. Then, find the column that most closely matches the pretest probability of streptococcal infection in this patient. The columns representing a typical pretest probability of strep throat for adults (12%) and children (33%) are in boldface.

		Pretest probability of strep throat								
No. of points	Likelihood ratio	5%	10%	**12%**	15%	20%	25%	**33%**	40%	50%
0	0.16	1	2	**2**	2	3	5	**7**	10	14
1	0.30	2	3	**4**	5	7	9	**13**	17	23
2	0.75	4	8	**9**	12	16	20	**27**	33	43
3	2.10	10	19	**22**	27	34	41	**51**	58	68
4	6.30	25	41	**46**	53	61	68	**76**	81	86

Let us consider various scenarios, with each assuming a 12% likelihood of strep throat for adults and 33% for children. If a child has cervical adenopathy, tonsilar exudate, a history of fever, and no cough, he gets 4 points. By going to the last row of the "33%" column, you see quickly that this corresponds to a 76% likelihood of streptococcal pharyngitis. It may be appropriate to treat him empirically with an antibiotic. An adult with none of the four cardinal characteristics gets 0 points and has a low likelihood of a streptococcal infection (approximately 2%). She can be managed with symptomatic therapy only. Finally, a child with fever, cough, and adenopathy but no exudate gets 2 points and has a 27% likelihood of streptococcal pharyngitis. This child could undergo further testing, perhaps using a rapid antigen screen, to refine the estimate of the likelihood of strep. With this information, a physician can deliver patient-centered care, individualized to the needs of each patient.

This book collects clinical prediction rules for use in the evidence-based practice of medicine. Slawson and Shaughnessy have described the usefulness of medical information as follows.[3]

$$\text{Usefulness of medical information} = \frac{\text{relevance} \times \text{validity}}{\text{work}}$$

Thus the most useful information is relevant to your patients, is valid, and requires little work to apply to your practice. This book addresses each element of usefulness for each clinical prediction rule. By reviewing the description of the patients, the setting, and the pretest probability of disease, you can decide if it is relevant to your practice. The study size, type of validation, and comments can help you evaluate the rule's validity. Most of the rules in this book have been validated in a new group of patients. Finally, by collecting all of the rules in one easy-to-use handbook and making software available, we reduce your work.

■ ORGANIZATION OF EACH CHAPTER

Not all clinical prediction rules are ready for immediate application to primary care practice. In some cases, a rule was developed at a tertiary care center and may not apply to the practice of community-based physicians. Other rules may not have been properly validated by testing their performance on patients distinct from those with whom they were developed. Still others use vague definitions of variables that are difficult to apply. In this book, we give you the information you need to apply clinical prediction rules rationally in your practice.

Each chapter describes the clinical rules for a group of related conditions, such as the circulatory system or infectious disease. Within each chapter, rules are divided into groups by symptom or diagnosis. Finally, each clinical prediction rule is presented in a structured, consistent fashion. The characteristics of each rule are discussed in more detail below.

1. *Clinical question:* This sentence describes the question the rule is attempting to answer.

2. *Population and setting:* Inclusion and exclusion criteria are used by researchers to describe the group of patients used to develop and validate the clinical rule. Criteria that are too restrictive may make the rule less generalizable; it may not apply to patients in the primary care setting if only patients with the most severe disease at a tertiary care center were included. On the other hand, broad inclusion criteria may adversely affect the accuracy of the rule; to paraphrase the old aphorism: The rule that tries to do everything does nothing.

Despite increasing interest in practice-based research, most studies still take place in academic medical centers and teaching hospitals. Patients in these settings tend to be sicker, typically present late in the course of an illness, and may undergo more intensive evaluation and monitoring than patients in the community setting. Even practice-based research may be biased by the fact that community physicians who participate in these studies may be more up-to-date, more motivated, or otherwise different from their colleagues who do not.

For example, a group of researchers developed a clinical prediction rule designed to identify patients with suspected myocardial infarction who are at high risk of dying. It uses findings from the initial electrocardiogram such as pathologic Q waves, left ventricular hypertrophy, and sustained ventricular tachycardia. In the university population in which the rule was developed, the risk of dying was 17 times higher in the high risk group than in the low risk group. However, when applied to a community hospital population, the risk was only 2.9 times higher.[4]

The same disease may present differently in different racial and ethnic groups. Once diagnosed, the prognosis may also vary between groups. For example, the prognosis of breast cancer and prostate cancer in black women and men is worse than that for a similarly aged group of white patients. A clinical prediction rule developed to predict the outcome of these diseases for white patients may therefore produce overly optimistic results when applied to a group of black patients. In an example from my own research, a clinical prediction rule developed to predict the outcome of cardiopulmonary resuscitation in hospitalized patients did not generalize well to African American patients in an urban setting.[5]

3. *Study size:* The size of the study group is an important indicator of study quality. All other things being equal, rules that have been tested in a large population are more likely to be valid than those validated in only a small group. In addition, rules that have been validated in several medical centers, hospitals, or practices are more likely to be generalizable to your patients than those tested in only a single setting.

4. *Pretest probability:* The prevalence of disease can affect the ability to transport a clinical prediction rule from one setting to another. This can happen when applying a clinical rule developed in the emergency room to the outpatient setting, or one developed in the intensive care unit to the general hospital ward. A rule developed in a setting where the prevalence of disease is 30% overestimates the likelihood disease when used in a group of patients with a prevalence of disease of only 10%. It is possible to adjust the rule for the new prevalence of disease using Bayes' theorem. However, the rule must be stated as a series of likelihood ratios, with a different likelihood ratio for each possible outcome of the rule.[6] We speak more about likelihood ratios below.

5. *Type of validation:* Validation is a key step in the development of a clinical prediction rule. If successful, it helps ensure clinicians that patients are properly classified by the rule. If not, it points out weaknesses of the rule and lays the groundwork for future research. Validation of a clinical prediction rule ideally involves testing the rule on a group of patients distinct from the group used to develop it. The group initially used to develop the rule is called the "training," or "derivation," group, and the group used to evaluate the rule is the "test," or "validation," group. The best validation procedures are prospective, where the validation takes place after the rule has been developed. Validation ideally takes place in one or more settings distinct from that in which the rule was initially developed. Finally, it is most convincing if the validation study is performed by a group of investigators other than those who originally developed the rule.

All of the above steps help minimize the possibility that selection, testing, and measurement biases do not adversely affect the generalizability of the clinical prediction rule. Unfortunately, such thorough validation procedures are rare. A summary of the approaches to validation is shown below (grade I is best, grade IV is worst):

Grade	Validation procedure
I	Validation group from a distinct population. The rule is developed in one group of patients and validated in another group, perhaps by a different group of researchers.
II	Split sample with prospective validation group. The data are gathered for the training group, the rule is developed, and it is then prospectively validated in the same location(s) by the same researchers.
III	Split-sample method. The patients are randomly divided into two groups, with one used to train the rule and one used to validate it.
IV	No validation or the training group was used as the validation group.

Most of the rules in this book have been prospectively validated (grade I or II). Although it does not guarantee that the rules are accurate in your setting with your patients, it does increase the likelihood that the results are valid and generalizable. When rules are poorly validated (grade III or IV), they should first be prospectively validated in your setting before applying them to the care of your patients.

6. *Comments:* The comments help put the rule in a clinical context. It is the section wherein any additional information important to rational application of the rule at the point of care is provided.

7. *Reference(s):* The reference(s) for the article describing the validation of this rule is given here. Rules that are more than 10–15 years old should be used only after careful consideration. Although some clinical measures have not changed (e.g., ST segment deviation on an electrocardiogram), others may be interpreted quite differently nowadays. For example, many patients who would have been hospitalized 20 years ago are now managed as outpatients. The length of stay is shorter, and criteria for certain diagnoses have changed with the widespread adoption of the ICD-9 codes. Thus it is imperative that early clinical prediction rules be carefully examined for the presence of such historical bias.

STATISTICS

Like any medical test, results of the validation procedure for a clinical prediction rule can be described using a number of statistics. The most commonly used are the sensitivity and specificity, the positive and negative predictive value, the likelihood ratio, the area under the receiver operating curve, and the misclassification rate. Each has advantages and disadvantages that are discussed in more detail below.

Sensitivity and Specificity

Sensitivity and specificity are the most widely used measures of the performance of medical tests, including clinical prediction rules. The definitions are as follows.

Sensitivity = the proportion of patients with disease who have a positive test

Specificity = the proportion of patients without disease who have a negative test

The major advantage of using sensitivity and specificity to describe the accuracy of a clinical prediction rule is the fact that these statistics do not change as the prevalence of disease changes. Their major limitation is that they assume we know whether the patient has the disease in question. As all clinicians know, though, we use a test (and a clinical prediction rule is a kind of test) because we do not know the actual disease state; we rely on the results of the test to guide our management. That is where predictive values and likelihood ratios come in.

Positive and Negative Predictive Values

More useful to clinicians in the real world are the positive and negative predictive values. They are defined as follows.

Positive predictive value = the proportion of patients with a positive test who actually have disease

Negative predictive value = the proportion of patients with a negative test who are actually free of disease

Although useful for a clinician trying to interpret the results of a clinical prediction rule, predictive values have a significant limitation. Unfortunately, the predictive values change as the likelihood of disease changes. Because many clinical prediction rules are developed in a population with a high prevalence of disease, they often have less impressive positive predictive values when used in the typical primary care setting, where the likelihood of disease is lower. On the other hand, the negative predictive value is improved by moving to a lower prevalence setting, although it does not increase as much as the positive predictive value decreases.

Consider the example of using the anti-nuclear antibody (ANA) to diagnose systemic lupus erythematosus (SLE). In a rheumatologist's office, where the likelihood of SLE in patients with joint pain is relatively high, the ANA has a fairly good positive predictive value. In the primary care setting, where SLE is rare, the positive predictive value is poor, but the negative predictive value is quite good.

Likelihood Ratios

The likelihood ratio (LR) associated with a positive test result describes the probability that a finding is present in diseased patients divided by the probability that it is present in nondiseased persons.[1] Put another way, the "posttest odds of disease" are equal to the "pretest odds of disease" multiplied by the likelihood ratio. These relations can be summarized with the following two equations.

$$\text{LR} = \frac{\text{probability that finding is present in patients with disease}}{\text{probability that finding is present in patients without disease}}$$

$$\text{Posttest odds} = \text{pretest odds} \times \text{LR}$$

If a test is simply positive or negative, one can calculate a likelihood ratio for a positive test result (LR^+) and a likelihood ratio for a negative test result (LR^-) using the sensitivity and specificity.

$$LR^+ = \text{sensitivity}/(100 - \text{specificity})$$

$$LR^- = (100 - \text{sensitivity})/\text{specificity}$$

Because the likelihood ratio can be calculated from the sensitivity and specificity, the likelihood ratio does not change as the prevalence of disease changes.

Likelihood ratios can also be calculated for multiple levels of positive. What does that mean? Consider the serum ferritin test, a test for iron-deficiency anemia (IDA). Although laboratories generally report a single cutoff value to indicate an abnormality, we know that as the serum ferritin increases the likelihood of IDA decreases. The likelihood ratio gives us a richer way to interpret the serum ferritin level, as shown in the table below.

Serum ferritin (mg/dl)	LR
≤15	51.8
15–24	8.8
25–34	2.5
35–44	1.8
45–100	0.5
≥100	0.08

Source: Sackett, Richardson, Rosenberg, Haynes. Evidence-Based Medicine: How to Practice and Teach EBM. Churchill Livingstone, London, 1997.

We use the same process for the creatinine kinase test for acute myocardial infarction, the CAGE score for alcoholism, the Strep Score, or any test that reports results as a continuous variable. If you want to know how to interpret a likelihood ratio, the following table gives some general guidelines:

Likelihood ratio	Interpretation
>10	Strong evidence to rule in disease
5–10	Moderate evidence to rule in disease
2–5	Weak evidence to rule in disease
0.5–2.0	No significant change in the likelihood of disease
0.2–0.5	Weak evidence to rule out disease
0.1–0.2	Moderate evidence to rule out disease
<0.1	Strong evidence to rule out disease

Source: Sackett, Richardson, Rosenberg, Haynes. Evidence-Based Medicine: How to Practice and Teach EBM. Churchill Livingstone, London, 1997.

The advantages of using likelihood ratios are significant. For example, if a clinical prediction rule results in a range of values from 0 to 4, the likelihood ratio for each level could be reported, giving the clinician more specific information. Also, because of the relation between pretest and posttest odds, it is easy to transport rules developed in one setting and apply them in another setting where the pretest odds of disease are either higher or lower.

By calculating likelihood ratios, you can also use a nomogram to convert the pretest probability to the posttest probability. See page 8 for an example.

Comparing Sensitivity, Specificity, Predictive Value, and Likelihood Ratios

The table below summarizes the characteristics of the sensitivity, specificity, predictive values, and likelihood ratios.

Test	Clinical value/meaning	Stability with changing prevalence	Can use multiple levels of a test result
Sensitivity or specificity	No	Yes	No
Predictive value	Yes	No	No
Likelihood ratio	Yes	Yes	Yes

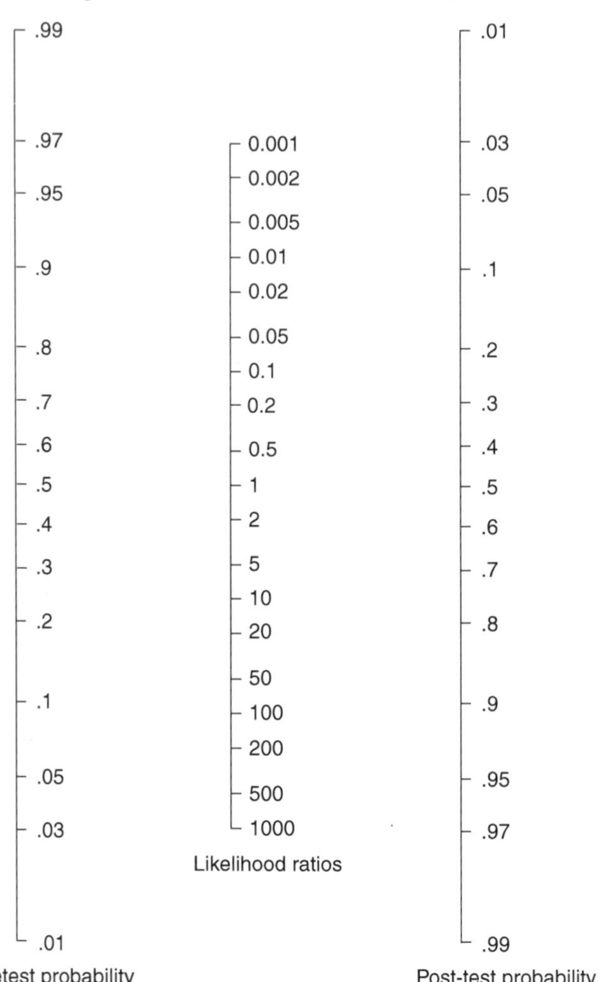

Thus the likelihood ratio is the only measure of test accuracy that has clinical relevance, does not change as the prevalence changes, and offers the ability to easily report multiple levels of "positivity" for a test.

Receiver-Operating Characteristic Curves

Receiver-operating characteristic (ROC) curves graph sensitivity on the y-axis and (100 − specificity) on the x-axis. The area under the ROC curve typically ranges from 0.5 (for a rule with no predictive power) to 1.0 (for a rule that perfectly categorizes all patients). A "good" rule typically has an area under the curve of at least 0.7, and an "excellent" rule has an area of more than 0.85. The area under the curve corresponds to the probability that a physician using the rule will correctly classify a pair of patients, one of whom has disease and one of whom does not.[7] A receiver-operating characteristic curve is shown below.

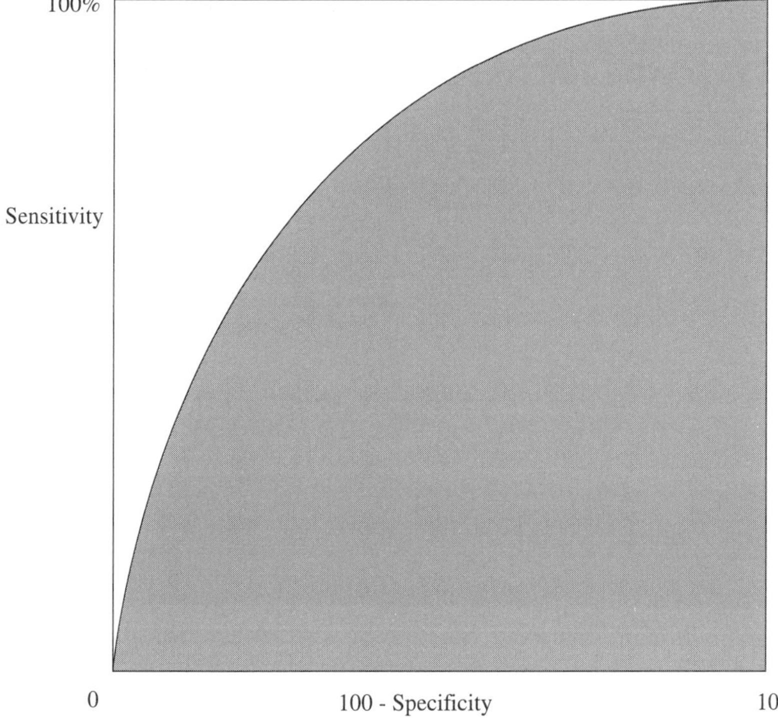

Although useful, the area under the ROC curve does not provide information about how patients are misclassified. For example, a rule with a high sensitivity but relatively low specificity may be useful for case-finding or screening, and one with low sensitivity and high specificity may be appropriate to "rule-in" disease. Nevertheless, both may have a fairly mediocre area under the ROC curve. Thus, in addition to reporting the area under the ROC curve, physicians should also utilize another measure of performance, such as likelihood ratios or predictive values.

An interesting feature of ROC curves is the slope: It is equal to the likelihood ratio. Thus while the curve is rising rapidly, the slope is positive and corresponds to a high likelihood ratio. As the curve flattens, the slope drops below 1 and corresponds to a decreased likelihood of disease.

Misclassification Rate

The misclassification rate is simply the number of patients misclassified by a rule divided by the total number of patients. Consider the figure below.

		Actual outcome	
		Disease	No disease
Predicted outcome	Disease	a	b
	No disease	c	d

Misclassification rate = (a+c) / (a+b+c+d)

Although the misclassification rate is useful, it does not tell us whether the misclassified patients were in cell b or c, which is important in some cases. For example, if a rule was designed to predict which patients with chest pain are having a myocardial infarction (MI), one would want to avoid false negatives (when the rule says a patient is not having an MI but they actually are). Therefore we would want few patients in cell c. On the other hand, if the rule makes a false-positive recommendation (cell b), the patient may be overtreated but is unlikely to suffer significant harm.

■ A FINAL NOTE

It is important to remember that any clinical diagnostic tool—whether a magnetic resonance imaging scan, a careful history, a blood test, or a clinical prediction rule—has limitations. The information in this book is intended to serve as an aid to the trained clinician for determining the diagnosis and prognosis of common medical conditions. The prediction, diagnosis, or prognosis of any of these rules is an estimate based on data from patients in another setting. *It simply tells us the probability of the outcome in question in a similar group of patients in some other city at some other time. It does not tell us with certainty whether **our patient** will have that outcome.* For example, when talking to a patient about prognosis, it may be helpful to frame the information this way: "For every 100 patients with symptoms like yours, about 50 will still be alive at 6 months. However, some live a lot longer, and some may not live as long as that."

The information in this book should never be a substitute for the considered judgment of the patient's personal physician in consultation with the patient, consultants, and all other information available. Slavish application of these clinical practice rules is inappropriate, potentially dangerous, and strongly discouraged. We encourage users to validate these rules carefully in their own setting before applying them to the care of their patients.

Finally, these rules can be excellent teaching tools. Beyond their clinical application, the rules tell us which clinical variables are particularly important or useful. For example, when diagnosing sinusitis we should make sure we know how to perform transillumination; and when diagnosing streptococcal pharyngitis it is important to pay attention to adenopathy, fever, exudate, and cough. They can also be the basis for practice-based research projects, particularly when the rules are not well validated (grade III or IV validation).

Any book like this is a work in progress. New rules are being developed all the time, and old favorites are being validated. If I missed one of your favorites, please let me know by sending an e-mail message to ebell@msu.edu. If you know of a better validation study, let me know as well. The National Library of Medicine does not have a separate indexing term for clinical rules, making it difficult to find them (which is why I wrote this book). I hope that by the time the next edition of this handbook appears, I will have many more well validated rules to include.

References

1. Sox HC, Blatt MA, Higgins MC, Marton KI. Medical Decision Making. Butterworth-Heinemann, Boston, 1988
2. Mark DB, Shaw L, Harrell FE, et al. Prognostic value of a treadmill exercise score in outpatients with suspected coronary artery disease. N Engl J Med 1991;325:849–853
3. Slawson DS, Shaughnessy AS. Becoming an information master: A guidebook to the medical information jungle. J Fam Pract 1994;39:593–594.
4. Young MJ, McMahon LF, Stross JK. Prediction rules for patients with suspected myocardial infarction. Arch Intern Med 1987; 147:1219–1222
5. Ebell MH, Kruse JA, Smith MA, Novak J, Wilcox J. Multivariate prediction: failure of three decision rules to predict the outcome of in-hospital cardiopulmonary resuscitation. Med Decis Making 1997;17:171–177
6. Poses RM, Cebul RD, Collins M, Fager SS. The importance of disease prevalence in transporting clinical prediction rules. Ann Intern Med 1986;105:586–591
7. Hanley JA, McNeil BJ. The meaning and use of the area under a receiver operating characteristic (ROC) curve. Radiology 1982;143:29–36.

2

Cardiovascular Disease

CHEST PAIN

Diagnosis of Acute Cardiac Ischemia Using the Acute Cardiac Ischemia–Time Insensitive Predictive Index (ACI-TIPI)

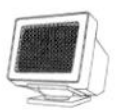

Clinical question

Which patients presenting to an emergency department with acute chest pain have acute cardiac ischemia (myocardial infarction, new onset angina, or unstable angina)?

Population and setting

Consecutive male patients over age 30 and female patients over age 40 presenting to the emergency room with one of the following chief complaints were included: chest pain, shortness of breath, upper abdominal pain, or dizziness. The settings were six New England hospitals (two university, two teaching, two nonteaching rural hospitals). The mean age was between 60.9 and 63.7 years (depending on the hospital); approximately 59% of patients were male and about 95% were white.

Study size

The training group had 3453 patients and the validation group 2320.

Pretest probability

In the training group, 19% had acute myocardial infarction, 17% had new-onset or unstable angina pectoris, and 64% had neither.

Type of validation

Grade II: The validation group was a separate sample from the same population, with data for the validation group gathered prospectively.

Comments

This is a widely used and well validated rule. It can be used as a clinical tool, although it is important to recall that the pretest probability of acute cardiac ischemia was quite high for the group used to develop the rule (36%).

Reference

Selker HP, Griffith JL, D'Agostino RB. A tool for judging coronary care unit admission appropriateness, valid for both real-time and retrospective use. Med Care 1991; 29:610–627.

CLINICAL PREDICTION RULE

1. Find your patient's clinical findings and associated values (x) and weights (b) below.

Variable	Weight (b_1)	Value (x_1)
Chest or left arm pressure or pain:present	1.231	1
Not present		0
Chest or left arm pain is chief complaint	0.882	1
Not chief complaint		0
Gender		
Male	0.712	1
Female		0
Age		
≤40 years	−1.441	1
>40 years		0
>50 years	0.667	1
≤50 years		0
Male patient more than 50 years old	−0.426	1
Otherwise		0
ECG Q waves 1 mm	0.616	1
Otherwise		0
ST segment		
Elevated 2 mm or more	1.314	2
Elevated 1–2 mm		1
Otherwise		0
ST segment (STDEP)		
Depressed 2 mm or more	0.993	2
Depressed 1–2 mm		1
Depressed 0.5–1.0 mm		0.5
Otherwise		0
T waves		
Hyperacute (50% QRS deviation)	1.095	1
Otherwise		0
T waves (TWINV)		
Inverted 5 mm or more	1.127	2
Inverted 1–5 mm		1
T waves flat		0.5
Otherwise		0
Both STDEP and TWINV not 0	−0.314	1
Otherwise		0

Note: ECG findings must be present in at least two leads; not due to block, LVH, or pacer; and T inversion in aV_R is excluded.

2. The probability of acute cardiac ischemia or ACI (myocardial infarction, new onset angina, or unstable angina) is calculated from these equations.

$$\text{Factor} = \exp(-3.933 + b_1x_1 + b_2x_2 + b_3x_3 + \ldots)$$

$$\text{Risk of ACI (\%)} = 100 \times [1 - 1/(1 + \text{factor})]$$

Example: A 53-year-old man with ST segment depression of 2.5 mm and chest pain as a chief complaint.

$$\text{Factor} = \exp[-3.933 + (1.231 \times 1) + (0.882 \times 1) + (0.712 \times 1) + (0.667 \times 1) + (0.993 \times 2)]$$

$$\text{Factor} = 4.6879$$

$$\text{Risk of ACI (\%)} = 100 \times [1 - 1/(1 + 4.6879)] = 82.4\%$$

Which Patients with Acute Chest Pain Require Intensive Care

Clinical question

Which patients with acute chest pain will have complications requiring intensive care?

Population and setting

The authors studied patients with a chief complaint of chest pain unexplained by local trauma or abnormality on the chest radiograph. The study took place in the three university hospitals and four community hospitals that participated in the Multicenter Chest Pain Study. In the validation group, 669 were age 30–39 years, 961 age 40–49 years, 975 age 50–59 years, and 2071 were over age 60; half were male.

Study size

The rule was developed using a group of 10,682 patients and tested in a group of 4676.

Pretest probability

Of these patients, 5.7% had a major event: ventricular fibrillation, cardiac arrest, new complete heart block, insertion of a temporary pacemaker, emergency cardioversion, cardiogenic shock, use of an intraaortic balloon pump, intubation, recurrent pain requiring coronary artery bypass graft (CABG), or percutaneous transluminal coronary angioplasty (PTCA).

Type of validation

Grade II: The test set was a separate sample from the same population, with data for the test set gathered prospectively.

Comments

This large, well designed study was developed from data at both community and university hospitals. It is well validated (prospectively) on a large validation group and has good predictive accuracy. In addition, the variables used in the rule are clear and unambiguous.

Reference

Goldman L, Cook EF, Johnson PA, et al. Prediction of the need for intensive care in patients who come to emergency departments with acute chest pain. N Engl J Med 1996;334:1498–1504.

CLINICAL PREDICTION RULE

1. Count the number of risk factors.

Variable	Points
Systolic blood pressure below 110 mm Hg	1
Rales heard above the bases bilaterally on physical examination	1
Known unstable ischemic heart disease, defined as a worsening of previously stable angina, new onset of postinfarction agina, angina after a coronary revascularization procedure, or pain that was the same as that associated with a previous MI	1
Total:	

2. Next, determine whether your patient is at very low risk, low risk, moderate risk, or high risk.

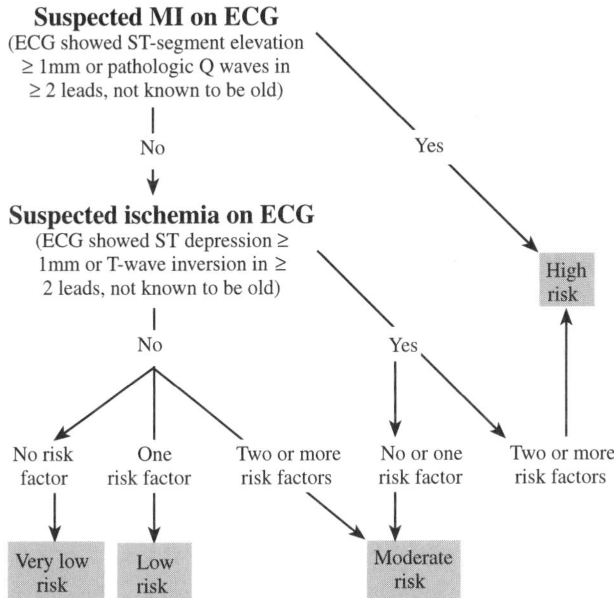

3. Based on the risk class, find your patient's *risk of a first major event* below (major events include ventricular fibrillation, cardiac arrest, new complete heart block, insertion of a temporary pacemaker, emergency cardioversion, cardiogenic shock, use of an intraaortic balloon pump, intubation, or recurrent pain requiring CABG or PTCA).

	Risk of a first major event (%)				
Risk class	<12 Hours	>12–24 Hours	>24–48 Hours	>48–72 Hours	0–72 Hours
High	7.6%	3.4%	3.2%	2.9%	16.1%
Moderate	1.1%	2.2%	2.7%	2.1%	7.8%
Low	0.5%	1.2%	1.1%	1.1%	3.9%
Very low	0.2%	0.2%	0.2%	0%	0.6%
Area under the ROC curve[a]	0.84	0.77	0.77	0.81	0.80

[a]ROC = receiver operating characteristics. An area of 1.0 indicates a perfect test, and an area of 0.5 indicates a worthless test.

Identification of Low-Risk Patients with Chest Pain

Clinical question

Based on elements of the history and physical examination alone, which patients are at very low risk for acute myocardial infarction (AMI) or unstable angina?

Population and setting

Consecutive patients age 25 or older who went to the Brigham and Women's emergency room in Boston with a chief complaint of chest pain unexplained by obvious local trauma or chest radiograph were included. The mean age was 56 years; 52% were women; and 53% were eventually admitted.

Study size

Altogether, 596 patients were studied.

Pretest probability

Eventually 17% were diagnosed with an AMI and another 24% with unstable angina. Diagnosis was based on standard enzyme and electrocardiographic (ECG) criteria if the patient was hospitalized. Of patients not hospitalized, 83% were reevaluated 3 days later in person and the remainder by telephone.

Type of validation

Grade IV: The training group was used as the validation group.

Comments

This rule should be used with great caution because it has not been prospectively validated. It would be especially helpful to validate it in the primary care office setting, as we are often faced with the evaluation of patients with chest pain, without access to rapid laboratory results or telemetry.

Reference

Lee TH, Cook EF, Weisberg M, Sargent RK, Wilson C, Goldman L. Acute chest pain in the emergency room: identification and examination of low risk patients. Arch Intern Med 1985;145: 65–69.

CLINICAL PREDICTION RULE

Low risk groups and their risk of acute myocardial infarction (MI) and unstable angina are shown below.

Clinical variable	No. of patients in this group	Acute MI	Unstable angina
Sharp or stabbing pain; no prior angina or MI	98	4%	2%
Sharp or stabbing pain; pain is pleuritic, positional, or reproduced by palpation	66	0%	3%
Sharp or stabbing pain; no prior angina or MI; pain is pleuritic, positional, or reproduced by palpation	48	0%	0%

Acute Chest Pain and Normal or Nonspecific ECG (Identification of Low-Risk Patients)

Clinical question

Among patients with acute chest pain and a normal or nonspecific ECG, what is the risk of acute myocardial infarction (AMI)?

Population and setting

Adult patients aged 30 years or older presenting to the emergency department with chest pain unexplained by obvious local trauma or chest radiograph abnormalities were included. Demographic information is not given.

Study size

The training group had 3495 patients and the validation group 1993 patients.

Pretest probability

Normal ECG: 3% had an AMI
Nonspecific ECG changes: 5% had an AMI

Type of validation

Grade II: The validation group was a separate sample from the same population, with data for the validation group gathered prospectively.

Comment

It is possible to identify a low risk group of patients who present with acute chest pain but have a normal or nonspecific ECG and no or few risk factors.

Reference

Rouan GW, Lee TH, Cook EF, Brand DA, Weisberg MC, Goldman L. Clinical characteristics and outcome of acute myocardial infarction in patients with initially normal of nonspecific electrocardiograms. Am J Cardiol 1989;64:1087–1092.

CLINICAL PREDICTION RULE

1. Read the ECG, and decide whether it is normal or has nonspecific changes. (*Note:* this clinical rule does not apply to clearly abnormal ECGs.)

Definitions

Normal: ECG is completely within normal limits without any ST or T wave abnormalities

Nonspecific changes: ECG has nonspecific ST or T wave changes, including minor ST or T wave abnormalities not suggestive of ischemia or strain

2. Count the number of risk factors your patient has.

Risk factor	Points
Age over 60 years	1
Male gender	1
Pain described as pressure	1
Pain radiating to arm, shoulder, neck, or jaw	1
Total:	

3. Determine your patient's risk of AMI for their number of points and type of ECG.

	Normal ECG		Nonspecific ECG	
Points	No. in group	With AMI	No. in group	With AMI
0	177	0%	114	0%
1	374	1.1%	309	2.6%
2	354	2.5%	333	4.8%
3	137	9.0%	149	11.0%
4	19	26.0%	26	23.0%

Ruling out Myocardial Infarction in 12 Hours

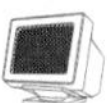

Clinical question

In which patients with acute chest pain can you effectively rule out myocardial infarction during a 12-hour period?

Population and setting

Patients over age 30 with acute anterior, precordial, or left-sided chest pain without obvious local trauma or abnormalities were studied at several community and university hospitals. The mean age was 62 years, and 58% were men.

Study size

A total of 2685 patients were used to validate the clinical rule.

Pretest probability

Altogether, 30% had an acute myocardial infarction (AMI), 28% unstable angina, and 42% other diagnoses.

Type of validation

Grade II: The test set was a separate sample from the same population, with data for the test set gathered prospectively.

Comments

This is a well validated rule established by experienced investigators who used a large validation group. Patients even came from a variety of settings, including community hospitals, improving the generalizability of the rule. It may be particularly valuable for use in the "chest pain centers" cropping up in emergency departments around the United States. Among patients who had a less than 7% risk of MI and who did not have either elevation of cardiac enzyme levels or recurrence of ischemic chest pain, only 4 of 771 had an MI.

Reference

Lee TH, Juarez G, Cook EF, et al. Ruling out acute myocardial infarction: a prospective multicenter validation of a 12-hour strategy for patients at low risk. N Engl J Med 1991;324:1239–1246.

CLINICAL PREDICTION RULE

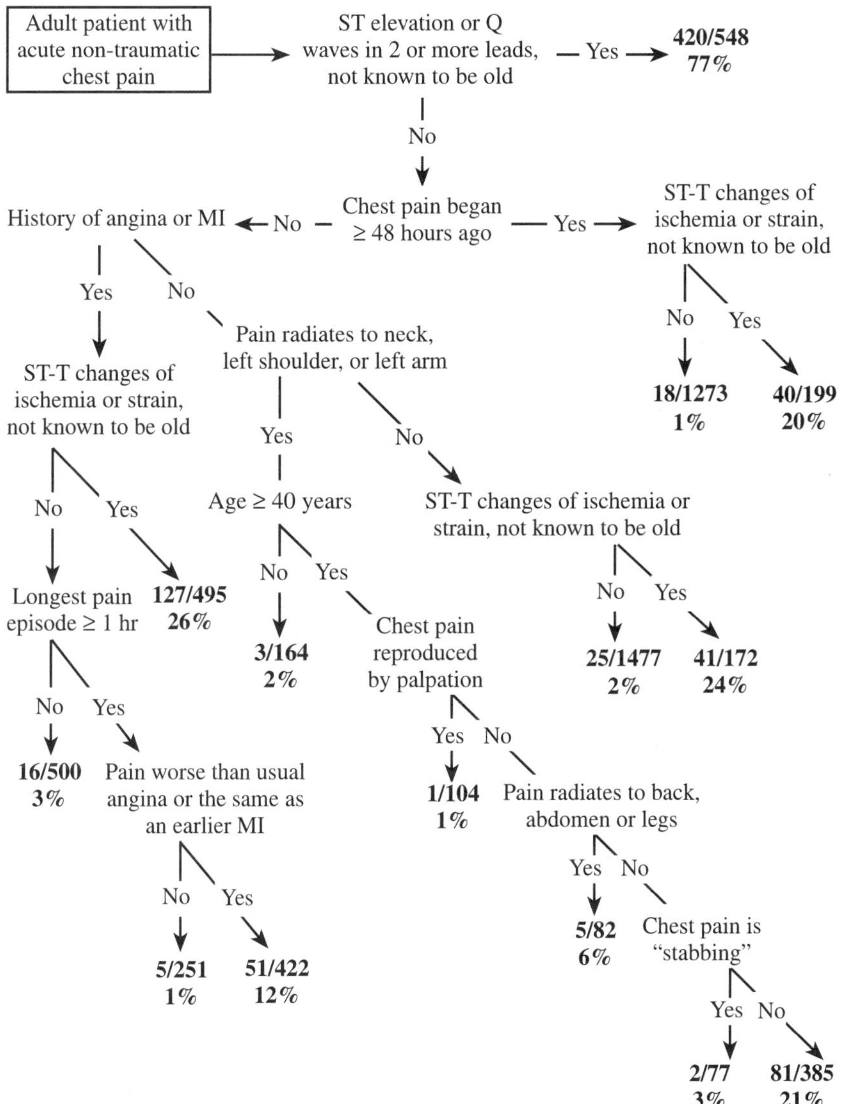

MYOCARDIAL INFARCTION

Diagnosis of Inferior Wall Myocardial Infarction

Clinical question

Which patients with chest pain have an inferior wall myocardial infarction (MI)?

Population and setting

Patients presenting to a university hospital with chest pain were included. Half had a normal coronary angiogram, half had an inferior MI based on a ventriculogram. The median age was 56 years in the inferior MI group (14% female) and 49 in the control group (57% female).

Study size

The training group had 432 patients and the validation group 236.

Pretest probability

Of the patients, 50% had an inferior MI (artificially generated due to the case–control design).

Type of validation

Grade III: The validation group was a separate sample from the same population, but data for both training and validation groups were gathered at the same time.

Comments

The authors used an adequate size validation group and split-sample validation, with clear definitions. However, the pretest probability is not calculable. The rule was developed by taking a group of patients without heart disease and a group with inferior MI and then finding the best set of variables to discriminate between the two. The rule is likely to be less effective when the likelihood of inferior MI is less than 50% (or more than 50%, for that matter); that is because, in general, tests work best when the likelihood of disease is exactly 50%.

Reference

Pahlm O, Case D, Howard G, Pope J, Haisty WK. Clinical prediction rules for ECG diagnosis of inferior myocardial infarction. Comp Biomed Res 1990;23:332–345.

CLINICAL PREDICTION RULE

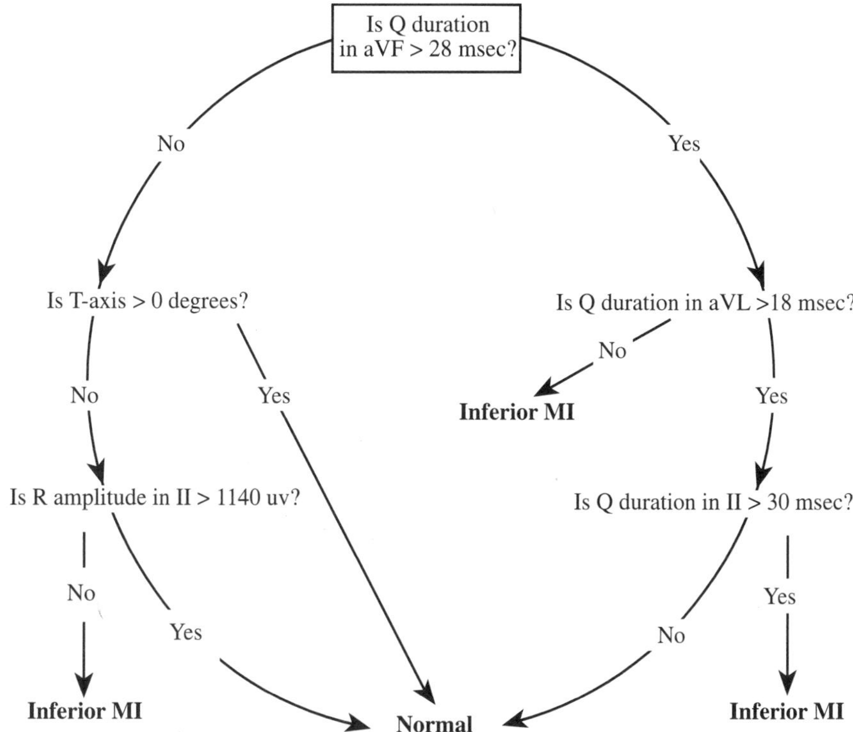

This diagram is 82% sensitive and 91% specific for the correct diagnosis of inferior MI (LR + 9.0, LR − 0.2).

Diagnosis of Myocardial Infarction in Patients with Left Bundle Branch Block

Clinical question

Which patients with acute chest pain and left bundle branch block (LBBB) have an acute myocardial infarction (AMI)?

Population and setting

Two groups of patients were included: those with AMI and LBBB from the GUSTO-1 trial, and a matched set of patients with unstable angina from the Duke Database of Cardiovascular Disease. The mean age was 68 years; 62% were male.

Study size

The training group had 262 patients and the validation group only 45.

Pretest probability

Of the patients, 50% had an MI (the training and validation groups were artificially derived to achieve a 50% disease prevalence).

Type of validation

Grade II: The validation group was a separate sample from the same population, with data for the validation group gathered prospectively.

Comments

The patients used to derive and validate this rule were taken from the GUSTO-1 trial and matched with a group of controls with unstable angina from a separate database. The 50% likelihood of disease makes the test look better than it probably is, so expect worse performance among groups of patients with a lower likelihood of LBBB. Also, the patients with LBBB were highly selected, having to meet fairly stringent criteria for the GUSTO-1 trial.

Reference

Sgarbossa EB, Pinski SL, Barbagelata A, et al. Electrocardiographic diagnosis of evolving acute myocardial infarction in the presence of left bundle-branch block. N Engl J Med 1996;334:481–487.

CLINICAL PREDICTION RULE

1. Add up the score for your patient.

ECG criterion	Odds ratio for acute MI (95% CI)	Score
ST segment elevation ≥ 1 mm and concordant with QRS complex	25.2 (11.6–54.7)	5
ST segment depression ≥ 1 mm in lead V_1, V_2, or V_3	6.0 (1.9–19.3)	3
ST segment elevation ≥ 5 mm and discordant with QRS complex	4.3 (1.8–10.6)	2
	Total:	

CI = confidence interval.

2. Find the percentage with MI in the table below (data from training group).

Score	No. with MI/total with that score
0	20/129 (16%)
2–3	15/27 (56%)
5	44/50 (88%)
7–8	48/52 (92%)
10	4/4 (100%)

3. From the validation group: A score of 3 or more has a sensitivity of 36% and specificity of 96% for the diagnosis of AMI in a patient with LBBB, with an area under the ROC curve of 0.87.

Diagnosis of Non-Q Wave MI

Clinical question

Which patients with chest pain, evidence of ischemia, and no Q waves have a non-Q wave myocardial infarction (MI) and which have unstable angina?

Population and setting

Patients with ischemic cardiac chest pain of between 5 minutes' and 6 hours' duration and objective evidence of ischemia [transient ST segment elevation (<30 minutes) or depression (≥0.1 mV) or T wave inversion, history of acute MI, or ≥70% stenosis on previous coronary angiogram] were included. Exclusion criteria included age ≥76, MI within the past 21 days, angioplasty within 6 months, pulmonary edema, previous CABG, cardiogenic shock, contraindications to thrombolytic therapy, and left bundle branch block. The average age was 58 years; 65% were male.

Study size

The training group had 735 patients and the validation group 735 patients.

Pretest probability

A non-Q wave MI was found in 33% of patients.

Type of validation

Grade III: The validation group was a separate sample from the same population, although data for both training and validation groups were gathered at the same time.

Comments

This study had an adequate size validation group, but the inclusion and exclusion criteria should be carefully examined before applying this rule to your patients. Also, "recent-onset angina" was not clearly defined and is left to your discretion.

Reference

Cannon CP, Thompson B, McCabe CH, et al. Predictors of non-Q-wave acute myocardial infarction in patients with acute ischemic syndromes: an analysis from the Thrombolysis in Myocardial Ischemia (TIMI) III trials. Am J Cardiol 1995;75:977–981.

CLINICAL PREDICTION RULE

1. Add up the number of risk factors for your patient.

Risk factor	Points
No prior angioplasty	1
Duration of pain ≥60 minutes	1
ST segment deviation	1
Recent-onset angina	1
Total:	

2. Find the probability of non-Q wave MI.

No. of risk factors	Probability of MI for a patient with this score
0	7.0%
1	19.6%
2	24.4%
3	49.9%
4	70.6%

Note: Data shown are for the training and validation groups combined. They were not reported separately but did not appear to be significantly different based on the description in the article.

Mortality Associated with Acute Myocardial Infarction

Clinical question

Which patients with acute myocardial infarction (AMI) will die?

Population and setting

Consecutive male patients over age 30 and female patients over age 40 presenting to the emergency room with an AMI were included. The settings were six New England hospitals (two university, two teaching, and two nonteaching rural hospitals). The mean age was 64 years; 64% were male.

Study size

The training group had 719 patients with AMI, and the validation group had 226.

Pretest probability

The mortality rate in the validation group was 14.3%.

Type of validation

Grade II: The validation group was a separate sample from the same population, with data for the validation group gathered prospectively.

Comments

This rule is a cousin to the ACI-TIPI (see above). It is probably most useful for comparing mortality rates among institutions.

Reference

Selker HP, Griffith JL, D'Agostino RB. A time-insensitive predictive instrument for acute myocardial infarction mortality: a multicenter study. Med Care 1991;29:1196–1211.

CLINICAL PREDICTION RULE

1. Find your patient's clinical findings and associated values (x) and weights (b) below.

Variable	Value (x_1)	Weight (b_1)
Age		
< 50 years	50	0.0733
50–80 years	Patient's age	
> 80 years	80	
Systolic BP (mm Hg)		
> 175	175	−0.0145
≤ 175	Patient's SBP	
Systolic BP (mm Hg)		
< 80	36	0.0347
80–140	$(140 - \text{SBP})^2/100$	
> 140	0	
T waves		
Peaked T waves present	2	0.6008
Inverted T waves present	1	
Otherwise	0	
Q waves		
Anterior-lateral Q waves	2	0.6453
Anterior-septal significant Q waves *or* anterior Q waves *or* poor R wave progression	1	
Otherwise	0	
Heart rate (mm Hg) < 110 *or* SVT present	0	0.7683
≤ 90 systolic blood pressure (mm Hg)	1	
91–110 systolic blood pressure	(SBP − 70)/20	
111–140 systolic blood pressure	2	
141–155 systolic blood pressure	(155 − SBP)/7.5	
> 155 systolic blood pressure	0	

Note: ECG findings must be present in at least two leads; not due to block, left ventricular hypertrophy, or pacer; and T inversion in aVR is excluded. SVT = supraventricular tachycardia; SBP = systolic blood pressure.

2. The probability of death for a patient with AMI is calculated using these formulas.

$$\text{Factor} = \exp(-5.6769 + b_1x_1 + b_2x_2 + b_3x_3 + \ldots)$$

$$\text{Risk of death with AMI (\%)} = 100 \times [1 - 1/(1 + \text{Factor})]$$

Example: A 53-year-old man with an initial systolic blood pressure of 157, a heart rate of 90, and anterior-lateral Q waves:

$$\text{Factor} = \exp[-5.6769 + (0.0733 \times 53) + (157 \times -0.0145) + (2 \times 0.6453)]$$

$$\text{Factor} = 0.062169$$

$$\text{Risk of death with AMI} = 100 \times [1 - 1/(1 + 0.062169)] = 5.85\%$$

Prognosis for AMI Based on Initial ECG

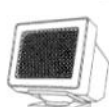

Clinical question

What is the prognosis for patients with acute myocardial infarction (AMI) based on their initial presentation and ECG?

Population and setting

Patients in the GUSTO-1 trial who presented within 6 hours of onset of chest pain were included. This study included more than 34,000 patients with AMI at 1081 hospitals around the world. The mean age was 61 years; 75% were male.

Study size

Altogether, 17,000 patients were in the training group, and 17,000 were in the validation group.

Pretest probability

Of all the patients, 6.8% died.

Type of validation

Grade III: The validation group was a separate sample from the same population, although data for both training and validation groups were gathered at the same time.

Comments

This large study provides some prognostic information based on the patient's initial presentation. It is limited by the fact that these patients were part of a clinical trial and therefore represent a relatively highly selected, closely monitored group, which may limit the generalizability of the rule to other populations.

Reference

Hathaway WR, Peterson ED, Wagner GS, et al. Prognostic significance of the initial ECG in patients with acute myocardial infarction. JAMA 1998;279:387–391.

CLINICAL PREDICTION RULE

1. Add up the points for your patient.

Risk factor	Points
Systolic blood pressure (mm Hg)	
40	46
50	40
60	34
70	28
80	23
90	17
100	11
110	6
>110	0
Pulse (beats/minute)	
40	0
60	0
80	6
100	11
120	17
140	23
160	28
180	34
200	40
Age (years)	
20	0
30	13
40	25
50	38
60	50
70	62
80	75
90	87
100	100
Height (cm)	
140	30
150	27
160	23
170	19
180	15
190	11
200	8
210	4
220	0
Killip class	
I	0
II	8
III	18
IV	30

Risk factor	Points
QRS duration (ms)	
Anterior MI	
60	16
80	21
100	26
120	31
140	36
160	41
180	47
200	52
Not anterior MI	
60	22
80	23
100	25
120	26
140	27
160	29
180	30
200	32
History of diabetes mellitus	6
ECG evidence of prior MI	10
Prior coronary artery bypass graft	10
No ECG evidence of prior MI and not AMI	10
Sum of absolute ST segment deviation (mm)	
0	0
10	7
20	15
30–70	19
80	18
Total:	

2. Find the corresponding probability of death.

Score	Mortality
0–74	0.1%
75–92	0.5%
93–104	1.0%
105–113	2.0%
114–119	3.0%
120–123	4.0%
124–127	5.0%
128–130	6.0%
131–132	7.0%
133–135	8.0%
136–137	9.0%
138–145	10.0%
146–158	20.0%
159–173	40.0%
174–188	60.0%
>188	80.0%

Diagnosis of Myocardial Infarction in the Emergency Department

Clinical question

Which patients in the emergency department with chest pain have a myocardial infarction (MI)?

Population and setting

All men aged 30 years and older and all women aged 40 and older who had a complaint of chest pain in the emergency department were enrolled. The mean age was 56 years.

Study size

There were 270 patients in the training group and 270 in the validation group.

Pretest probability

Altogether, 34% had myocardial infarction

Type of validation

Grade III: The validation group was a separate sample from the same population, although data for both training and validation groups were gathered at the same time.

Comments

This well designed clinical prediction rule has adequate validation group size, definitions, and fairly good validation. Importantly, there were few inclusion/exclusion criteria, making it more likely to apply to your patients. The rate of MI was on the high side, at 34%, though. The outcome is most useful with a very low or very high score; a risk of MI of 1.8% may still be too high for physicians to be comfortable discharging a patient without careful informed consent; but it can still be useful for deciding whether step-down unit or intensive care unit admission is warranted.

Reference

Tierney WM, Roth BJ, Psaty B, et al. Predictors of myocardial infarction in emergency room patients. Crit Care Med 1985;13:526–531.

CLINICAL PREDICTION RULE

1. Add up the risk factors for your patient.

Risk factor	Points
ST elevation ≥ 1 mm in at least one lead (old, new, or unknown)	1
New Q wave (> 40 ms in duration or > than one-third the height of R wave)	1
Diaphoresis with chest pain	1
Past history of MI	1
Total:	

2. Find your patient's risk of acute MI.

No. of risk factors present	No. with MI/total
0	5/278 (1.8%)
1	8/161 (5.0%)
2	22/67 (32.8%)
3 or 4	22/27 (79.4%)

Note: These results are for both derivation and validation groups; there was little difference in the area under the ROC curve between the two groups. Results were not reported for the validation group alone in the original article.

HEART MURMURS

Evaluation of a Systolic Murmur

Clinical question

Which patients with a systolic murmur need an echocardiogram?

Population and setting

Patients aged 18–55 years referred for echocardiography to evaluate a systolic murmur at an urban general internal medicine clinic were included. Patients were excluded if they had a prior diagnosis of coronary artery disease, cardiomyopathy, valvular disorders, valve replacement, or endocarditis; if they had undergone prior echocardiography; if they were an inpatient; or if they were referred to rule out endocarditis.

Study size

There were 102 patients in the study.

Pretest probability

A positive echocardiogram was seen in 39.2%.

Type of validation

Grade IV: The training group was used as the validation group.

Comments

This small study has several limitations but was included because it is the only clinical prediction rule addressing this relatively common clinical question. The most important problems are the lack of an independent validation group and the small size of the training and validation groups. It should be used only with great caution. However, the definitions are precise and reproducible, and the statistical methodology is appropriate. It is also highly questionable whether physicians and patients would be satisfied with a negative predictive value of 88% in young women with a low grade murmur (i.e., 12% would still have a clinically important murmur).

Reference

Fink JC, Schmid CH, Selker HP. A decision aid for referring patients with systolic murmurs for echocardiography. J Gen Intern Med 1994;9:479–484.

CLINICAL PREDICTION RULE

Probability of a significant murmur =

$$\frac{1}{(1 + \exp[-\{-3.65 + (0.074 \times \text{age}) + (1.77 \times \text{gender}) + (1.61 \times \text{grade})\}])}$$

where age is in years; gender: 1 if male, 0 if female; and grade = 1 if the murmur is ≥ 3/6 and 0 if the murmur is < 3/6.

Not ordering echocardiograms for women 35 years and younger with murmur grades ≤ 2 would have 90% sensitivity and 47% specificity (4/33 had a positive murmur compared with 36/69 of all other patients), with a positive predictive value of 48% and negative predictive value of 88%.

Predictors of Survival after Aortic Valvuloplasty

Clinical question

What is the likelihood of event-free survival among patients who have undergone balloon aortic valvuloplasty?

Population and setting

Consecutive patients undergoing balloon aortic valvuloplasty for symptomatic aortic stenosis were studied. The mean age was 78 years; 44% were male. Most had congestive heart failure (CHF) (82%); 36% had angina and 25% syncope. Coronary artery disease was absent in 54%, and 41% had a left ventricular ejection fraction under 50%.

Study size

Altogether, 205 patients were studied.

Pretest probability

The probability of event-free survival (defined as survival without recurrent symptoms, repeated valvuloplasty, or aortic valve replacement) was 18% over the mean follow-up period of 2 years.

Type of validation

Grade IV: The training group was used as the validation group.

Comments

Most patients had an event by the end of the 2-year follow-up period. At highest risk were patients with a low aortic systolic pressure, those with a high pulmonary capillary wedge pressure, and those with the smallest decrease in peak aortic valve gradient after surgery. This rule should be used with great caution, as it has not been prospectively validated.

Reference

Kuntz RE, Tosteson AN, Berman AD, et al. Predictors of event-free survival after balloon aortic valvuloplasty. N Engl J Med 1991;325:17–23.

CLINICAL PREDICTION RULE

1. Gather the following data for your patient:
   Percentage decrease in peak aortic-valve gradient (pAVG) after surgery: ___%
   Mean pulmonary capillary wedge pressure (PCWP) before angioplasty ___ mm Hg
   Mean aortic systolic pressure (AOSP) before angioplasty ___ mm Hg

2. Find the rate of event-free survival at 6, 12, 18, and 24 months corresponding to these values below.

	Before valvuloplasty		Event-free survival (%)			
Decrease in pAVG	PCWP (mm Hg)	AOSP (mm Hg)	At 6 months	At 12 months	At 18 months	At 24 months
≥55%	<18	≥140	87	79	69	59
		110–139	83	72	58	48
		<110	76	61	46	34
	18–25	≥140	83	73	60	49
		110–139	78	64	49	37
		<110	69	52	35	24
	>25	≥140	79	66	51	40
		110–139	72	56	39	28
		<110	62	43	26	15
40–54%	<18	≥140	85	76	64	54
		110–139	80	68	54	42
		<110	73	57	40	28
	18–25	≥140	81	69	55	34
		110–139	75	60	44	32
		<110	65	47	30	19
	>25	≥140	76	62	46	34
		110–139	68	51	34	23
		<110	57	37	21	11
<40%	<18	≥140	79	66	51	39
		110–139	72	56	39	27
		<110	62	42	25	15
	18–25	≥140	73	57	41	29
		110–139	64	46	29	18
		<110	52	32	16	8
	>25	≥140	66	48	31	20
		110–139	56	36	20	11
		<110	43	23	9	4

Aortic Stenosis and Aortic Valve Replacement

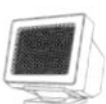

Clinical question

Which patients with aortic stenosis need aortic valve replacement?

Population and setting

Consecutive adult patients at a university hospital undergoing heart catheterization for suspected aortic stenosis were included. The mean age was 69 years (range 33–87 years). Diagnoses included congenital bicuspid valve ($m = 26$), rheumatic disease ($m = 6$), and degenerative calcific stenosis ($m = 71$).

Study size

The training group had 26 patients and the validation group 77.

Pretest probability

Aortic valve replacement was required in 76.6%.

Type of validation

Grade II: The validation group was a separate sample from the same population, with data for the validation group gathered prospectively.

Comments

This study is unusual in having a much larger validation group than training group, and validation did use a prospective methodology. The researchers followed patients for a year and used the data to predict which patients would eventually need a valve replacement. The rule discriminated well between patients who did and did not require valve replacement and should be useful to physicians despite the small sample size. Because the outcome is the need for surgery 1 year later, there is some potential for bias.

Reference

Otto CM, Pearlman AS. Doppler echocardiography in adults with symptomatic aortic stenosis. Arch Intern Med 1988;148:2553–2560.

CLINICAL PREDICTION RULE

Definitions

Vmax = maximum aortic jet velocity

Doppler AVA = Doppler aortic valve area

AI severity = aortic insufficiency severity (0 = absent, 1 + = turbulence localized adjacent to the aortic leaflets, 2+ = turbulence extending to the mitral valve leaflet tips)

AVR = aortic valve replacement

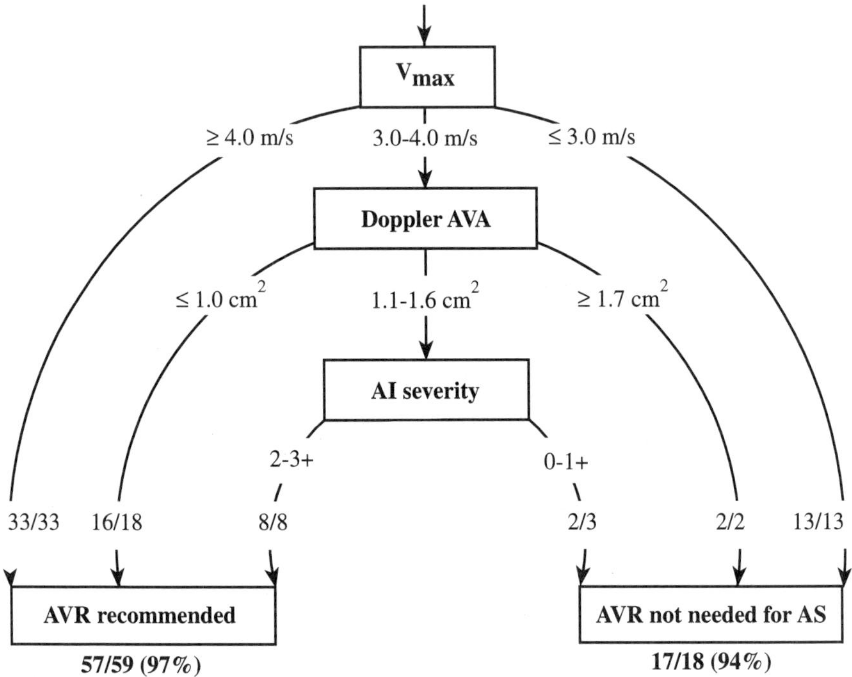

Among patients with AVR recommended by the rule, 57 of 59 (97%) needed aortic valve replacement; among those in whom AVR was not recommended, 17 of 18 (94%) did not require it.

PERIPHERAL VASCULAR DISEASE

Diagnosis of Peripheral Vascular Disease: Edinburgh Claudication Questionnaire

Clinical question

Which patients with leg complaints have intermittent claudication?

Population and setting

There were two groups in the validation group: 300 community patients seen in general practice with a mean age of 70 years and 50 vascular clinic patients with a mean age of 62 years. The latter group was included to "enrich" the sample with more patients who had intermittent claudication.

Study size

The training group had 647 patients; the validation group included 50 vascular clinic patients and 300 community patients.

Pretest probability

The prevalence of intermittent claudication was 7.4% in the community sample and 58% in the vascular clinic sample.

Type of validation

Grade II: The validation group was a separate sample from the same population, with data for the validation group gathered prospectively.

Comments

The diagnosis of intermittent claudication was made by clinicians, without any clear reference standard for the diagnosis or requirement for noninvasive testing.

Reference

Leng GC, Fowkes FG. The Edinburgh Claudication Questionnaire: an improved version of the WHO/Rose Questionnaire for use in epidemiological surveys. J Clin Epidemiol 1992;45:1101–1109.

CLINICAL PREDICTION RULE

Ask patients the following question:

1. Do you get a pain or discomfort in your legs when you walk? **Yes** □ No □

If you answered "Yes" to question 1, please answer the following questions.

2. Does this pain ever begin when you are standing still or sitting? Yes □ **No** □
3. Do you get it if you walk uphill or hurry? **Yes** □ No □
4. Do you get it when you walk at an ordinary pace on the level? Yes □ No □
5. What happens to it if you stand still?
   Usually continues more than 10 minutes □
   Usually disappears in 10 minutes or less □
6. Where do you get this pain or discomfort? Mark the place(s) with "x" on the diagram below

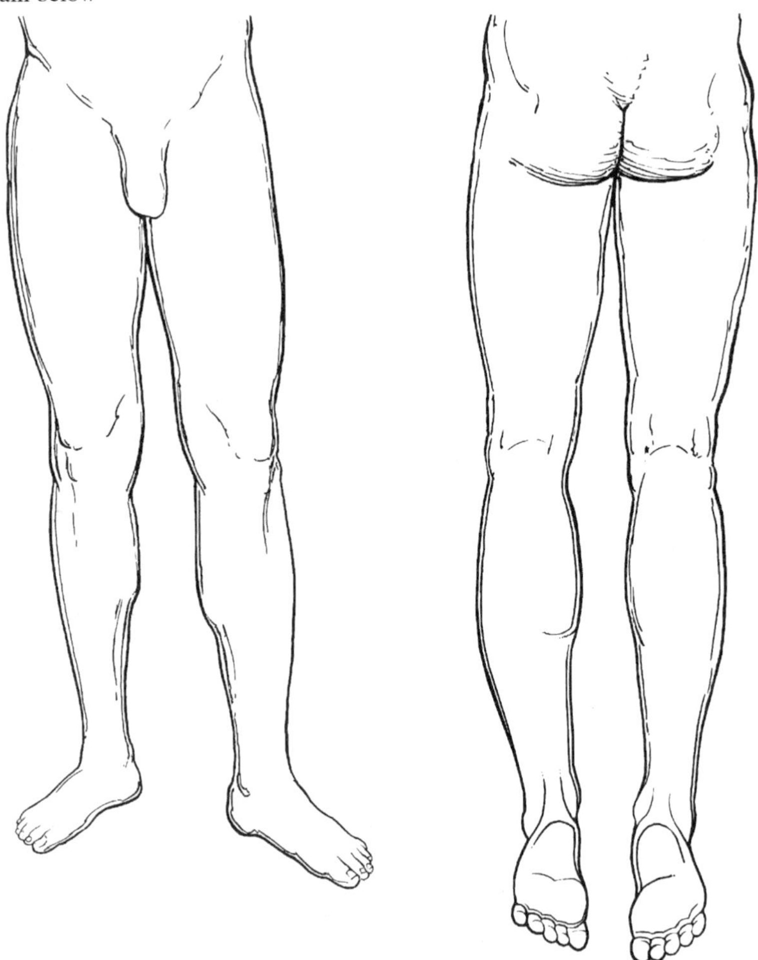

Interpreting the results of the questions: The diagnosis of *claudication* requires all of the following responses: "Yes" to 1, "No" to 2, "Yes" to 3, and "usually disappears in 10 minutes or less" to 5 (these responses are shown in boldface above). Grade 1 = "No" to 4 and Grade 2 = "Yes" to 4. If these criteria are fulfilled, a *definite claudicant* is one who indicates pain in the calf, regardless of whether pain is also marked in other sites. *Atypical claudication* is diagnosed if pain is indicated in the thigh or buttock, in the absence of calf pain. Subjects should not be considered to have claudication if pain is indicated in the hamstrings, feet, shins, or joints or appears to radiate, in the absence of pain in the calf.

This survey is 91% sensitive and 99% specific for the diagnosis of intermittent claudication.

CEREBROVASCULAR DISEASE

Risk of Stroke (Framingham Study)

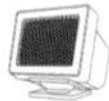

Clinical question

What is the risk of stroke during the next 10 years?

Population and setting

Patients age 30–74 from Framingham, Massachusetts who were part of the Framingham Heart Study were followed longitudinally for at least 12 years.

Study size

Altogether, 2590 persons were studied.

Pretest probability

The likelihood of stroke was 5.9% in men age 55–59 years and 3.0% in women 55–59 years; 11% in men 65–69 years and 7.2% in women 65–69 years; and 22.3% in men 80–84 years and 23.9% in women 80–84 years.

Type of validation

Grade IV: The training group was used as the validation group.

Comments

Although not prospectively validated, the otherwise good methods, long follow-up, and representativeness of the population make it a useful clinical rule.

Reference

Anderson KM, Wilson PW, Odell PM, Kannel WB. An updated coronary risk profile: a statement for health professionals. Am Heart J 1991;83:356–362.

CLINICAL PREDICTION RULE

1. Find the number of points for each risk factor in the six tables below.

Age (years)	Points
54–56	0
57–59	1
60–62	2
63–65	3
66–68	4
69–71	5
72–74	6
75–77	7
78–80	8
81–83	9
84–86	10

SBP if male (mm Hg)	Points
95–105	0
106–116	1
117–126	2
127–137	3
138–148	4
149–159	5
160–170	6
171–181	7
182–191	8
192–202	9
203–213	10

SBP if female (mm Hg)	Points
95–104	0
105–114	1
115–124	2
125–134	3
135–144	4
145–154	5
155–164	6
165–174	7
175–184	8
185–194	9
195–204	10

Htn Rx (women): add more points depending on the SBP level

SBP (mm Hg)	Points
95–104	6
105–114	5
115–124	5
125–134	4
135–144	3
145–154	3
155–164	2
165–174	1
175–184	1
185–194	0
195–204	0

For men, add points depending on risk factors

Risk factor	Points
Htn Rx	2
Cigarettes	3
Atrial fib	4
Diabetes	2
CVD	3
LVH	6

For women, add points depending on risk factors

Risk factor	Points
Htn Rx	See table at left
Cigarettes	3
Atrial fib	6
Diabetes	3
CVD	2
LVH	4

SBP = systolic blood pressure; Diabetes = history of diabetes? Htn Rx = under antihypertensive therapy? Cigarettes = smokes cigarettes? Atrial fib = history of atrial fibrillation? LVH = left ventricular hypertrophy on ECG? CVD = history of myocardial infarction, angina pectoris, coronary insufficiency, intermittent claudication, or congestive heart failure?

2. Add the points for all risk factors.

$$\frac{\quad}{\text{Age}} + \frac{\quad}{\text{SBP}} + \frac{\quad}{\text{Hyp Rx}} + \frac{\quad}{\text{Diabetes}} + \frac{\quad}{\text{Cigarettes}}$$

$$+ \frac{\quad}{\text{CVD}} + \frac{\quad}{\text{AF}} + \frac{\quad}{\text{LVH}} = \frac{\quad}{\text{Total}}$$

3. Find the risk corresponding to the point total.

	10-Year risk of stroke	
Points	Men	Women
1	2.6%	1.1%
2	3.0%	1.3%
3	3.5%	1.6%
4	4.0%	2.0%
5	4.7%	2.4%
6	5.4%	2.9%
7	6.3%	3.5%
8	7.3%	4.3%
9	8.4%	5.2%
10	9.7%	6.3%
11	11.2%	7.6%
12	12.9%	9.2%
13	14.8%	11.1%
14	17.0%	13.3%
15	19.5%	16.0%
16	22.4%	19.1%
17	25.5%	22.8%
18	29.0%	27.0%
19	32.9%	31.9%
20	37.1%	37.3%
21	41.7%	43.4%
22	46.6%	50.0%
23	51.8%	57.0%
24	57.3%	64.2%
25	62.8%	71.4%
26	68.4%	78.2%
27	73.8%	84.4%
28	79.0%	
29	83.7%	
30	87.9%	

4. Compare with the average 10-year risk of stroke.

	Risk of stroke	
Age (years)	Men	Women
55–59	5.9%	3.0%
60–64	7.8%	4.7%
65–69	11.0%	7.2%
70–74	13.7%	10.9%
75–79	18.0%	15.5%
80–84	22.3%	23.9%

Likelihood of Benefit from Carotid Endarterectomy

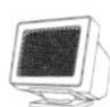

Clinical question

Which patients with a 70–99% carotid artery stenosis undergoing carotid endarterectomy are likely to benefit from surgery?

Population and setting

Patients with a carotid-distribution transient ischemic attack (TIA), minor stroke, non-disabling major stroke, or retinal infarct during the last 6 months and evidence of ipsilateral carotid stenosis were recruited for the European Carotid Surgery Trial.

Study size

The training group had 2060 patients and the validation group 990.

Pretest probability

The probability of an ipsilateral carotid territory major ischemic stroke, surgical major stroke, or death was 13% during the 5-year follow-up period.

Type of validation

Grade I: The validation group was from a distinct population. The rule was developed in one group of patients and validated in a separate group.

Comments

Data from patients with a 0–69% stenosis were used to develop a predictive model, which was then validated in the group with a 70–99% stenosis. Variables that predicted increased risk with medical management only were given positive point scores; those that predicted increased risk of death with endarterectomy were given negative point scores.

Reference

Rothwell PM, Warlow CP, European Carotid Surgery Trialists' Collaborative Group. Prediction of benefit from carotid endarterectomy in individual patients: a risk-modeling study. Lancet 1999;353:2105–2110.

CLINICAL PREDICTION RULE

1. Count up the points for your patient with a 70–99% carotid stenosis (range 0–5 points).

Risk factor	Medical risk points
Cerebral (not an ocular) event	1
Plaque surface irregularity	1
Any events[a] within the past 2 months	1
Degree of carotid stenosis	
70–79%	0
80–89%	1
90–99%	2
Total:	

[a]Carotid-distribution TIA, minor ischemic stroke, nondisabling major ischemic stroke, or a retinal infarction.

2. The 5-year risk of ipsilateral carotid territory ischemic stroke with optimal medical therapy is as follows.

Medical risk points	Patients	Strokes	5-Year risk of stroke (95% CI)
0	7	0	0%
1	48	2	6% (0–14%)
2	141	14	13% (7–20%)
3	123	22	21% (13–29%)
4	63	21	45% (31–60%)
5	12	4	38% (9–68%)

3. Next, determine the risk of surgical complications (any major stroke or death during the 30 days after surgery). Count up the points for your patient (range 0–3 points).

Risk factor	Surgical risk points
Female patient	1
Peripheral vascular disease (claudication or previous peripheral vascular surgery for ischemia)	1
Systolic blood pressure > 180 mm Hg	1
Total:	

4. The 30-day risk of any major stroke or death after carotid endarterectomy is as follows.

Surgical risk points	Patients (no.)	Strokes or deaths (no.)	30-Day risk of major stroke or death (95% CI)
0	238	14	4.7% (2.6–7.6%)
1	234	17	7.3% (4.3–11%)
2–3	64	8	12.5% (5.6–23%)

5. Now calculate the overall risk score to assist in decision-making regarding medical versus surgical treatment of 70–99% carotid stenosis in patients with symptoms during the previous 6 months (range 1.5–5 points).

Risk factor	Overall risk points
Cerebral (not ocular) event	1
Plaque surface irregularity	1
Any events[a] within the past 2 months	1
Degree of carotid stenosis	
70–79%	0
80–89%	1
90–99%	2
Female patient	−0.5
Peripheral vascular disease (claudication or previous peripheral vascular surgery for ischemia)	−0.5
Systolic blood pressure > 180 mm Hg	−0.5
Total:	

[a]Carotid-distribution TIA, minor ischemic stroke, nondisabling major ischemic stroke, or a retinal infarction.

6. The following table shows the outcomes for patients with either 0–3.5 or 4–5 overall risk points. Only patients with 4 or more overall risk points derive clinically significant benefit from surgery.

	5-Year risk of an adverse outcome[a]			
Overall risk points	Surgical treatment	Medical treatment	Absolute risk reduction with surgical treatment	NNT to prevent one adverse outcome
0–3.5	11%	12%	1%	100
4–5	7%	40%	33%	3
Total	10%	17%	7%	14

[a]Ipsilateral carotid territory major ischemic stroke, surgical major stroke, or death.
NNT = number needed to treat (i.e., you would have to treat 100, 3, or 14 patients, respectively, with surgery to prevent one adverse outcome.)

G-Score: Prognosis for Acute Stroke

Clinical question

What is the 6-month prognosis for patients with acute stroke?

Population and setting

Consecutive patients admitted with acute stroke during a 1-year period were included. The mean age was 73 years. Scores were calculated 24 hours after admission.

Study size

Altogether, 361 patients were enrolled in the validation group; and data were complete for 314 at 6 months.

Pretest probability

At 6 months, 39% had died and 29% were disabled.

Type of validation

Grade I: The validation group was from a distinct population. The rule was developed in one group of patients and validated in another.

Comments

This is a well designed study with adequate follow-up and prospective design in an independent population. The G-Score is a simplification of Guy's Score but was found to be nearly as accurate in this study.

Reference

Gompertz P, Pound P, Ebrahim S. Predicting stroke outcome: Guy's prognostic score in practice. J Neurol Neurosurg Psychiatry 1994;57:932–935.

CLINICAL PREDICTION RULE

1. Calculate the G-score at 24 hours after admission for acute stroke.

Variable	Points
Complete paralysis of worst limb	1
Hemiplegia + hemianopia + higher cerebral dysfunction[a]	1
Drowsy or comatose after 24 hours	1
Loss of consciousness at onset	1
Age (years)	
≤50	1
51–75	2
>75	3
Uncomplicated hemiparesis	−1
Total:	

[a]Higher cerebral dysfunction means dysphasia, perceptual, or cognitive impairment.

2. Find the patient's risk of a bad outcome (death or inability to walk independently).

G-score	No. with bad outcome	No. with good outcome	95% CI for percent with bad outcome	Likelihood ratio for bad outcome
≤2	39	44	36–58%	0.40
3	22	18	45–70%	0.55
4	36	22	60–74%	0.74
5	48	10	73–93%	2.2
≥6	71	4	90–100%	8.1

3. If you have additional information based on your setting or patient population to calculate the overall pretest risk of bad outcome, you can use the following table to refine your estimate.

	Prior probability of a bad outcome					
G-Score	40%	50%	60%	70%	80%	90%
≤2	21%	29%	38%	48%	62%	78%
3	27%	36%	45%	56%	69%	83%
4	33%	43%	53%	63%	75%	87%
5	59%	69%	77%	84%	90%	95%
≥6	84%	89%	92%	95%	97%	99%

Barthel Index for Stroke Rehabilitation

Clinical question

What is the prognosis for a patient with stroke?

Population and setting

The population of patients with acute stroke studied had an age range of 20–88 years, with a mean age of 69 years. Of the strokes, 47% were thrombotic, 14% hemorrhagic, 8% embolic, and 31% unknown.

Study size

Altogether, 110 patients were studied.

Pretest probability

Of the group, 80% returned to their homes.

Type of validation

Grade I: The test set was from a distinct population. The rule was developed in one group of patients and validated in another.

Comments

This is an early study of an even earlier clinical prediction rule first developed during the 1950s. Newer validations are needed, given the changes in patient care since 1979, so use these results with caution.

Reference

Granger CV, Dewis LS, Peters NC, et al. Stroke rehabilitation: analysis of repeated Barthel Index measures. Arch Phys Med Rehabil 1979;60:14–17.

CLINICAL PREDICTION RULE

1. Add up the points for your patient.

Item	Description	Points
Feeding	Independent. Able to apply any necessary device. Feeds in reasonable time.	10
	Needs help (i.e., for cutting).	5
Bathing	Performs without assistance.	5
Personal toilet (grooming)	Washes face, combs hair, brushes teeth, shaves (manages plug if electric razor).	5
Dressing	Independent. Ties shoes, fastens fasteners, applies braces.	10
	Needs help but does at least half of task in reasonable time.	5
Bowel control	No accidents. Able to use enema or suppository, if needed.	10
	Occasional accidents or needs help with enema or suppository.	5
Bladder control	No accidents. Able to care for collecting device if used.	10
	Occasional accidents or needs help with device.	5
Toilet transfers	Independent with toilet or bedpan. Handles clothes, wipes, flushes, or cleans pan.	10
	Needs help for balance, handling clothes, or toilet paper.	5
Chair/bed transfers	Independent, including locks of wheelchair and lifting footrests.	15
	Minimum assistance or supervision.	10
	Able to sit but needs maximum assistance to transfer.	5
Ambulation	Independent for 50 yards; may use assistive devices, except for rolling walker.	15
	With help for 50 yards.	10
	Independent with wheelchair for 50 yards, only if unable to walk.	5
Stair climbing	Independent. May use assistive devices.	10
	Needs help or supervision.	5
	Total:	

2. Interpretation.

Barthel score on admission	Discharged to hospital or nursing home	Discharged home
5–40	36%	64%
45–60	10%	90%
65–100	4%	96%

	Independence				Total dependence		
Barthel score on admission	Stairs	Ambulation	Chair/bed transfer	Dressing	Bowel	Grooming	Feeding
100	100%	100%	100%	100%	0%	0%	0%
85	0%	35%	76%	87%	0%	0%	0%
60	0%	0%	0%	3%	8%	0%	0%
40	0%	0%	0%	0%	67%	16%	0%
0	0%	0%	0%	0%	100%	100%	100%

CORONARY ARTERY DISEASE

Probability of CAD in Patients with Normal Resting ECG

Clinical question

What is the probability of coronary artery disease in patients with a normal resting electrocardiogram (ECG)?

Population and setting

All patients were referred for evaluation of suspected coronary artery disease (CAD) to undergo exercise testing or coronary angiography. Only those who eventually underwent coronary angiography within 3 months of exercise testing were included. Patients with known CAD were excluded. The training group was recruited between 1981 and 1993, and the validation group was recruited between 1993 and 1996. The mean age was 54 years; 46% were women.

Study size

The training group had 915 patients and the validation group 348.

Pretest probability

Altogether, 43% had significant CAD (at least one vessel with ≥ 50% obstruction), and 22% had severe CAD (two or more vessels with ≥70% obstruction).

Type of validation

Grade II: The test set was a separate sample from the same population, with data for the test set gathered prospectively.

Comments

This is a simple, well validated rule. It can help identify patients at high risk of significant or severe CAD who should undergo more urgent evaluation. It is especially useful in settings where access to catheterization is limited. This rule was developed and validated in a high risk population of patients, all of whom underwent coronary catheterization. Ideally, though, this rule should be validated prospectively in a low risk population. The probability of CAD in an unselected primary care population of patients with chest pain is much lower at all risk levels.

Reference

Morise AP, Haddad J, Beckner D. Development and validation of a clinical score to estimate the probability of coronary artery disease in men and women presenting with suspected coronary artery disease. Am J Med 1997;102:350–356.

CLINICAL PREDICTION RULE

1. Calculate the patient's risk score.

Variable	Points
Men's age (years)	
>55	9
40–55	6
<40	3
Women's age (years)	
>65	9
50–65	6
<50	3
Symptoms	
Typical angina	5
Atypical angina	3
Non-anginal	1
Estrogen status	
Premenopausal or on estrogen replacement	−3
Postmenopausal and not on estrogen replacement	+3
Male/unknown	0
Diabetes	2
Hypertension	1
Smoking	1
Hyperlipidemia	1
Family history of CAD (first-degree relative under age 60)	1
Obesity (body mass index > 27)	1
Total:	

2. Interpret the risk of CAD from the table below.

		Significant disease		Severe disease	
Risk score	Status	Men	Women	Men	Women
0–8	Low	15%	16%	5%	9%
9–15	Intermediate	49%	32%	28%	15%
16–24	High	67%	71%	52%	31%

Interpretation of Graded Exercise Tests

Clinical question

What is the pretest probability of coronary artery disease (CAD) for patients being referred for a graded exercise test?

Population and setting

The rule was developed from 211 patients with episodic chest pain admitted between November 1979 and November 1980 to Stanford University Medical Center for elective coronary arteriography. Demographic data are not available.

Study size

The training group had 211 patients and the validation group had 693, of whom 404 were self-referred from a VA population and 289 were self-referred from a Kaiser Permanente health maintenance organization.

Pretest probability

The clinical rule takes into account the pretest probability. The pretest probability was 76% in the training group.

Type of validation

Grade I: The validation group was from a distinct population. The rule was developed in one group of patients and validated in another.

Comments

This rule was validated in two populations. Likelihood ratios were calculated by the author of this book for each of the validation groups. A "mean" likelihood ratio is reported below.

Reference

Sox HC, Hickam DH, Marton KI, et al. Using the patient's history to estimate the probability of coronary artery disease: a comparison of primary care and referral practices. Am J Med 1990;89:7–14.

CLINICAL PREDICTION RULE

1. Calculate your patient's risk score from the risk factors below.

Risk factor	Points
Age > 60 years	3
Pain brought on by exertion	4
Patient must stop all activities when pain occurs	3
History of myocardial infarction	4
Pain relieved within 3 minutes of taking nitroglycerin	2
At least 20 pack-years of cigarette smoking	4
Male gender	5
Total:	

2. Find your patient's risk of CAD below, based on the pretest probability of disease.

		VA self-referred		Kaiser self-referred	
Score	Likelihood ratio[a]	No.	CAD	No.	CAD
0–4	0.01[b]	4	0%	98	0%
5–9	0.4	148	6%	125	6%
10–14	0.9	126	21%	39	10%
15–19	5	90	71%	20	30%
20–25	46	36	92%	7	86%
	Total:	404	33%	289	8%

[a]The likelihood ratios were calculated from the VA and Kaiser self-referred populations, taking a mean of the values for the two groups.

[b]The likelihood ratio of 0 for the score 0–4 was changed to 0.01 to facilitate more realistic calculations.

[c]Probability of CAD.

Probability of Complications after Coronary Angioplasty

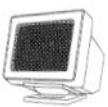

Clinical question

What is the likelihood of major complications [emergent coronary artery bypass grafting (CABG), myocardial infarction (MI), death] following coronary angioplasty?

Population and setting

Patients were recruited from 42 centers (76% community-based institutions) participating in a national angioplasty registry in 1992 (training group) and 1993 (validation group). Patients undergoing angioplasty for whom multivessel disease status was known (approximately half of the total population in the registry) were included. The mean age was 62 years.

Study size

There were 4289 patients in the training group and 5250 in the validation group.

Pretest probability

There was a 2.0% rate of major complications (death, emergent CABG, MI).

Type of validation

Grade II: The validation group was a separate sample from the same population, with data for the validation group gathered prospectively.

Comments

This well designed prediction rule used a large population, good definitions, and appropriate validation. It is useful for stratifying patients for closer than usual follow-up after angioplasty, but it does not necessarily predict long-term outcomes.

Reference

Kimmel SE, Berlin JA, Strom BL, et al. Development and validation of a simplified predictive index for major complications in contemporary percutaneous transluminal coronary angioplasty practice. J Am Coll Cardiol 1995;26:931–938.

CLINICAL PREDICTION RULE

1. Count how many of the following risk factors your patient has.

Risk factor	Points
Aortic valve disease (any aortic valve regurgitation or stenosis)	1
Left main coronary angioplasty	1
Shock (unsupported SBP < 80 mm Hg with a heart rate > 95 beats/min, peripheral signs of vascular collapse; includes patients on ventilator or intraaortic balloon pump or taking high doses of vasopressor agents; or patients receiving CPR)	1
Acute myocardial infarction within 24 hours before coronary angioplasty	1
Type C lesion coronary angioplasty	1
Multivessel disease (two or more lesions in two or more coronary distributions, each with ≥ 70% stenosis)	1
Unstable angina (crescendo angina despite medical therapy, postinfarction angina, or admitting diagnosis of unstable angina)	1
Total:	

SBP = systolic blood pressure; CPR = cardiopulmonary resuscitation.

2. Predict the outcome based on the number of risk factors present (overall complication rate was 2.0%).

No. of risk factors	Complication rate	Likelihood ratio
0	1.3% (2054)[a]	0.6
1–2	2.5% (2970)	1.1
3	5.4% (184)	2.5
> 3	16.7% (42)	8.7

[a]Number in the group.

Likelihood of Severe Coronary Artery Disease

Clinical question

What is the likelihood that a patient referred for cardiac catheterization has severe coronary artery disease (CAD)?

Population and setting

The population studied was consecutive adult patients referred to a university hospital for cardiac catheterization.

Study size

The training group had 6435 patients and the validation group 2342 patients.

Pretest probability

Altogether, 68% had significant coronary artery disease.

Type of validation

Grade II: The validation group was a separate sample from the same population, with data for the validation group gathered prospectively.

Comments

This is an important clinical question, and the rule is well validated with clear definitions. However, calculation requires use of exponentiation and a logistic equation, making it difficult to apply at the bedside without a computer or calculator. A nomogram is provided to help apply this rule.

Reference

Pryor DB, Shaw L, Harrell FE, et al. Estimating the likelihood of severe coronary artery disease. Am J Med 1991;90:553–562.

CLINICAL PREDICTION RULE

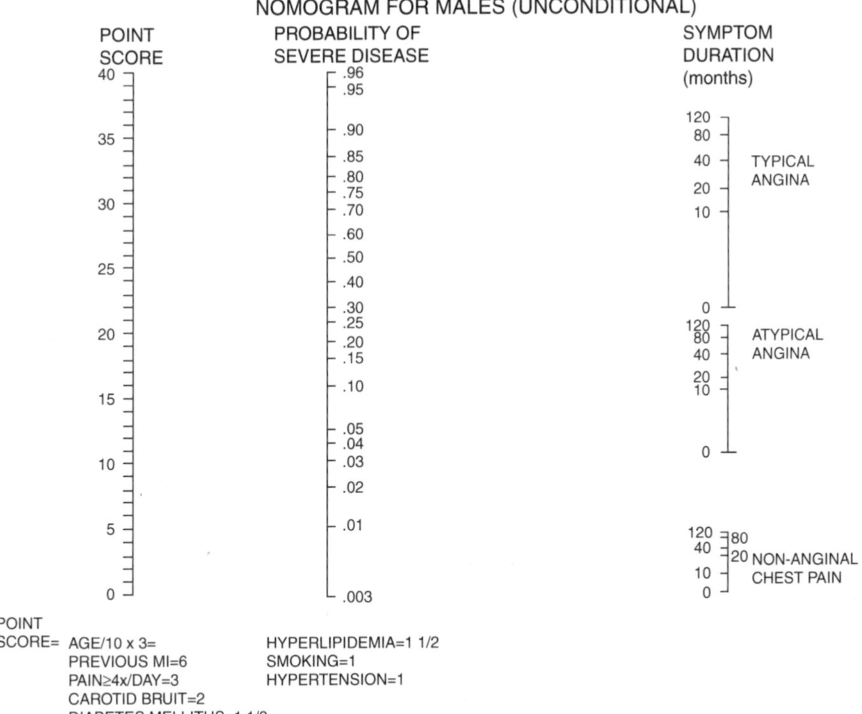

From Pryor DB, Shaw L, Harrell FE, et al. Estimating the likelihood of severe coronary artery disease. Am J Med 1991;90:553–562. Reproduced with permission.

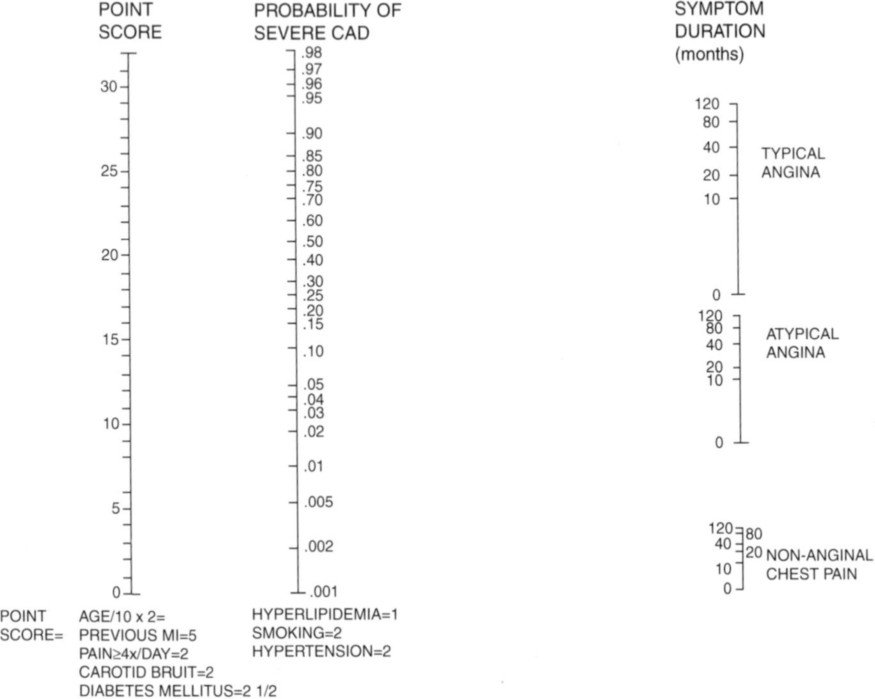

From Pryor DB, Shaw L, Harrell FE, et al. Estimating the likelihood of severe coronary artery disease. Am J Med 1991;90:553–562. Reproduced with permission.

In-hospital Mortality in Coronary Artery Bypass Surgery

Clinical question

What is the likelihood of in-hospital mortality after coronary artery bypass graft (CABG) surgery?

Population and setting

All patients undergoing CABG in Maine, New Hampshire, and Vermont between July 1987 and April 1989 were included.

Study size

There were 1539 patients in the training group and 1516 in the validation group.

Pretest probability

The in-hospital mortality rate was 4.3%

Type of validation

Grade III: The validation group was a separate sample from the same population, although data for both training and validation groups were gathered at the same time.

Comment

This study used a simple split-sample validation, but the large sample size and the fact that it is based on data from every hospital in two states makes it generalizable. Because of the rule's complexity and the need for exponentiation, it is best used with a computer or spreadsheet.

Reference

O'Connor GT, Plume SK, Olmstead EM, et al. Multivariate prediction of in-hospital mortality associated with coronary artery bypass graft surgery. Circulation 1992; 85:2110–2118.

CLINICAL PREDICTION RULE

1. First calculate the Charlson co-morbidity index.

Co-morbid condition	Points
Peripheral vascular disease	1
Chronic lung disease	1
Dementia	1
Chronic liver disease/cirrhosis	1
Preexisting peptic ulcer disease	1
Diabetes mellitus with no sequelae	1
Diabetes mellitus with end-organ sequelae	2
Preexisting renal disease	2
Leukemia, lymphoma, or solid cancer	2
Liver disease with sequelae	3
Metastatic or multiple cancers	6
Charlson Co-morbidity Index:	

2. Then multiply the cofactor in column A matching your patient by the coefficient in column B.

Variables	Column A	Column B	Subtotals
Age	Years	0.056	
Gender	0 = Male	0.278	
	1 = Female		
Body surface area (BSA)	$(BSA)^{0.5}$	−4.021	
Charlson Co-morbidity Index	0 = 0	0.381	
	1 = 1		
	2 = 2 or more		
Prior CABG	0 = No	1.288	
	1 = Yes		
Ejection fraction score	6 = ≥60%	0.095	
	10 = 50–59%		
	12 = 40–49%		
	14 = <40%		
LVEDP (mm Hg)	1 = ≤14	0.236	
	2 = 15–18		
	3 = 19–22		
	4 = >22		
Priority at surgery	1 = Elective	0.726	
	2 = Urgent		
	3 = Emergency		
Constant	1 for all patients	−4.374	
		Total:	

CABG = coronary artery bypass graft; LVEDP = left ventricular end-diastolic pressure.

3. Use the logistic regression model to predict the risk of in-hospital mortality.
   a. Calculate the odds using the patient's values and the coefficients from the regression equation.

$$\text{Odds} = \exp[-4.374 + (0.056 \times \text{age}) + (0.278 \times \text{gender}) + (-4.021 \times \sqrt{\text{BSA}}) + (0.381 \times \text{co-morbidity score}) + (1.288 \times \text{prior CABG}) + (0.095 \times \text{ejection-fraction score}) + (0.236 \times \text{LVEDP quartile}) + (0.726 \times \text{priority at surgery})]$$

b. Use the odds to calculate the predicted probability of in-hospital mortality:

$$\text{Probability} = \text{odds}/(1 + \text{odds})$$

4. Finally, find your patient's mortality.

Risk category	Observed mortality (95% CI)
<1.5%	0.3% (0–1.5%)
1.5–2.4%	1.0% (0.2–2.8%)
2.5–3.4%	3.6% (1.6–6.9%)
3.5–6.4%	4.5% (2.5–7.4%)
≥6.5%	12.5% (9.1–16.7%)

Coronary Artery Disease Risk (Framingham Study)

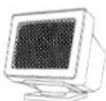

Clinical question

What is the risk of developing coronary heart disease during the next 5–10 years?

Population and setting

Patients age 30–74 from Framingham, Massachusetts who were part of the Framingham Heart Study were followed longitudinally for at least 12 years.

Study size

Altogether, 2590 persons were studied.

Pretest probability

The incidence of coronary heart disease was 5% in patients age 30–39 years, 11% in those 40–49 years, 20% in those 50–59 years, 29% in those 60–69 years, and 26% in those 70–74 years.

Type of validation

Grade IV: The training group was used as the validation group.

Comments

Although not prospectively validated, the otherwise good methods, long follow-up, and representativeness of the population make this clinical rule useful.

Reference

Anderson KM, Wilson PW, Odell PM, Kannel WB. An updated coronary risk profile: a statement for health professionals. Am Heart J 1991;83:356–362

CLINICAL PREDICTION RULE

1. Find the number of points for each risk factor in the six tables below.

Age if female (years)	Points
30	−12
31	−11
32	−9
33	−8
34	−6
35	−5
36	−4
37	−3
38	−2
39	−1
40	0
41	1
42–43	2
44	3
45–46	4
47–48	5
49–50	6
51–52	7
53–55	8
56–60	9
61–67	10
68–74	11

Age if male (years)	Points
30	−2
31	−1
32–33	0
34	1
35–36	2
37–38	3
39	4
40–41	5
42–43	6
44–45	7
46–47	8
48–49	9
50–51	10
52–54	11
55–56	12
57–59	13
60–61	14
62–64	15
65–67	16
68–70	17
71–73	18
74	19

HDL-cholesterol (mg/dl)	Points
25–26	7
27–29	6
30–32	5
33–35	4
36–38	3
39–42	2
43–46	1
47–50	0
51–55	−1
56–60	−2
61–66	−3
67–73	−4
74–80	−5
81–87	−6
88–96	−7

Total cholesterol (mg/dl)	Points
139–151	−3
152–166	−2
167–182	−1
183–199	0
200–219	1
220–239	2
240–262	3
263–288	4
289–315	5
316–330	6

SBP (mm Hg)	Points
98–104	−2
105–112	−1
113–120	0
121–129	1
130–139	2
140–149	3
150–160	4
161–172	5
173–185	6

Other factors	Points
Cigarettes[a]	4
Diabetes[b]	
Male gender	3
Female gender	6
ECG-LVH[c]	9

[a]Smokes cigarettes?
[b]Diabetes = history of diabetes?
[c]ECG-LVG = left ventricular hypertrophy on ECG?

2. Add the points for all risk factors.

$$\frac{}{\text{Age}} + \frac{}{\text{total chol}} + \frac{}{\text{HDL}} + \frac{}{\text{SBP}} + \frac{}{\text{smoking}}$$

$$+ \frac{}{\text{diabetes}} + \frac{}{\text{ECG-LVH}} = \frac{}{\text{total}}$$

3. Find the risk corresponding to the point total.

Points	Probability (%) 5 years	Probability (%) 10 years
≤1	<1	<2
2	1	2
3	1	2
4	1	2
5	1	3
6	1	3
7	1	4
8	2	4
9	2	5
10	2	6
11	3	6
12	3	7
13	3	8
14	4	9
15	5	10
16	5	12
17	6	13
18	7	14
19	8	16
20	8	18
21	9	19
22	11	21
23	12	23
24	13	25
25	14	27
26	16	29
27	17	31
28	19	33
29	20	36
30	22	38
31	24	40
32	25	42

4. Compare with average 10-year risk.

Age (years)	Probability (%) Women	Probability (%) Men
30–34	<1	3
35–39	<1	5
40–44	2	6
45–49	5	10
50–54	8	14
55–59	12	16
60–64	13	21
65–69	9	30
70–74	12	24

Duke Treadmill Score (Interpretation of Graded Exercise Testing)

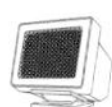

Clinical question

What is the long-term outcome for patients undergoing graded exercise testing?

Population and setting

Mark et al: Consecutive outpatients referred for evaluation of suspected coronary artery disease (CAD) to the Duke University Department of Cardiology who had a treadmill test were included. The median age was 54 (range 45–62 years); 67% were male. *Kwok et al:* Symptomatic patients who were referred for exercise thallium testing between 1989 and 1991; 939 had nonspecific ST-T wave changes on the resting ECG; 1466 had normal resting ECGs. The mean age was 62; 58% were male.

Study size

The validation group for outpatients included 613 patients and for inpatients 1428.

Pretest probability

Overall rates of 4-year survival were 92% for inpatients and 97% for outpatients.

Type of validation

Grade I: The validation group was from a distinct population. The rule was developed in one group of patients and validated in another. The results of two separate validations are given.

Comments

The Treadmill Score helps physicians interpret the results of a graded exercise test. Patients with a low risk of death over the next 4 years (those with a score of 5 or higher) are unlikely to benefit from aggressive interventions or surgery; they should be managed medically. Patients with a high likelihood of death (especially those with a score of less than −11) are more likely to benefit from an interventional approach. A limitation to this rule is that the population used to develop and evaluate it was already highly selected, with a higher rate of CAD than patients in the typical primary care population. Note that in the second validation study a distinction was made between patients with a normal resting ECG and those with nonspecific ST-T wave changes.

References

Kwok JM, Miller TD, Christian TF, Hodge DO, Gibbons RJ. Prognostic value of a treadmill exercise score in symptomatic patients with nonspecific ST-T abnormalities on resting ECG. JAMA 1999;282:1047–1053.

Mark DB, Shaw L, Harrell FE, et al. Prognostic value of a treadmill exercise score in outpatients with suspected coronary artery disease. N Engl J Med 1991;325:849–853.

CLINICAL PREDICTION RULE

1. Calculate the treadmill score.

Variable	Points
Duration of exercise in minutes	___ minutes
Maximal ST segment deviation during exercise	−5 × _____ mm
Angina index	
Exercise-limiting angina	−8
Nonlimiting angina	−4
No pain	−0
Total points:	

Note: Another way to calculate the score is using an equation:

Score = duration in minutes − (5 × ST deviation in mm) − (angina index)

2. Interpret the Duke Treadmill Score using the original data (Mark et al).

		4-Year survival rate	
Score	Risk group	Inpatients	Outpatients
+5 to +15	Low	98%	99%
−10 to +4	Intermediate	92%	95%
−25 to −11	High	79%	79%

3. Interpret the Duke Treadmill Score using a second validation (Kwok et al). Note that these patients were symptomatic and were referred for exercise thallium testing. Two sets of data are shown, one for patients with a normal resting ECG, and one for those with nonspecific ST-T wave changes.

	7-Year survival rate (%)		
Duke Treadmill Score	Overall mortality	Cardiac death	Cardiac death, AMI, or late revascularization
Normal resting ECG			
+5 to +15	95%	99%	88%
−10 to +4	91%	97%	78%
−25 to −12	78%	93%	60%
Resting ECG: NSSTTWC			
+5 to +15	91%	97%	84%
−10 to +4	80%	92%	73%
−25 to −12	78%	76%	38%

NSSTTWC = nonspecific ST-T wave changes; AMI = acute myocardial infarction.

Likelihood of Significant Coronary Artery Disease Using the History and Physical Examination

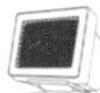

Clinical question

What is the likelihood that a patient referred for noninvasive testing has significant coronary artery disease (CAD)?

Population and setting

Consecutive, symptomatic patients referred for outpatient noninvasive testing at a university medical center ($n = 1030$) who subsequently underwent cardiac catheterization ($n = 168$) were studied.

Study size

There were 168 patients in the validation group.

Pretest probability

Of the 168 patients who underwent catheterization, 64.9% had significant CAD, 26.8% had severe disease, and 7.1% had left main CAD.

Type of validation

Grade I: The validation group was from a distinct population. The rule was developed in one group of patients and validated in another.

Comments

This question is important clinically, and the rule is well validated with clear definitions. However, calculation requires use of exponentiation and a logistic equation, making it difficult to apply at the bedside without a computer or calculator.

Reference

Pryor DB, Shaw L, McCants CB, et al. Value of the history and physical in identifying patients at increased risk for coronary artery disease. Ann Intern Med 1993;118:81–90.

CLINICAL PREDICTION RULE

Definitions

The variables in the equation (female gender, typical angina, atypical angina, history of myocardial infarction (MI), electrocardiogram (ECG) Q waves, hyperlipidemia, diabetes, ECG ST-T wave changes, and smoking) are graded 1 if present and 0 if absent.

1. Calculate x.

$$\begin{aligned} x = & -7.376 + (\text{age} \times 0.1126) - (0.328 \times \text{female}) - (0.0301 \times \text{age} \times \text{female}) \\ & + (2.581 \times \text{typical angina}) + (0.976 \times \text{atypical angina}) \\ & + (1.093 \times \text{history of MI}) + (1.213 \times \text{ECG Q waves}) \\ & + (0.741 \times \text{history of MI} \times \text{Q waves}) + (2.596 \times \text{smoking}) \\ & + (1.845 \times \text{hyperlipidemia}) + (0.694 \times \text{diabetes}) \\ & + (0.637 \times \text{ECG ST-T wave changes}) - (0.0404 \times \text{age} \times \text{smoking}) \\ & - (0.0251 \times \text{age} \times \text{hyperlipidemia}) + (0.550 \times \text{female} \times \text{smoking}) \end{aligned}$$

2. Estimate the probability of significant CAD (defined as at least 75% narrowing of a major coronary artery).

$$\text{Probability} = 1/(1 + e^{-x})$$

Likelihood of Left Main Coronary Artery Disease Using the History and Physical Examination

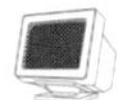

Clinical question

What is the likelihood that a patient referred for noninvasive testing has left main coronary artery disease (CAD)?

Population and setting

Consecutive, symptomatic patients referred for outpatient noninvasive testing at a university medical center ($n = 1030$) who subsequently underwent cardiac catheterization ($n = 168$) were studied.

Study size

There were 168 patients in the validation group.

Pretest probability

Of the 168 patients who underwent catheterization, 64.9% had significant CAD, 26.8% had severe disease, and 7.1% had left main CAD.

Comments

This question is important clinically, and the rule is well validated with clear definitions. However, calculation requires use of exponentiation and a logistic equation, making it difficult to apply at the bedside without a computer or calculator. Consider using Rule Retriever software to apply this rule.

Reference

Pryor DB, Shaw L, McCants CB, et al. Value of the history and physical in identifying patients at increased risk for coronary artery disease. Ann Intern Med 1993;118:81–90.

CLINICAL PREDICTION RULE

Definitions

Female is graded 1 if present, 0 if absent.

Typical angina is graded 1 if present, 0 if absent.

Vascular Disease Index is 1 point for each of the following (range 0–3).

History of peripheral vascular disease
History of cerebrovascular disease
Presence of carotid bruits

1. Calculate x:

$$x = -6.7271 + (1.1252 \times \text{typical angina}) + (0.0483 \times \text{age, maximum 65 years}) - (0.5770 \times \text{female}) + (0.5923 \times \text{Vascular Disease Index}) + [0.4027 \times \log_{10} (\text{duration of CAD in months} + 1)]$$

2. Estimate the probability of left main CAD.

$$\text{Probability} = 1/(1 + e^{-x})$$

■ ABDOMINAL AORTIC ANEURYSM

Perioperative Mortality for Abdominal Aortic Aneurysm

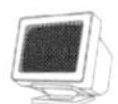

Clinical question

What is the perioperative mortality for patients undergoing elective surgery for abdominal aortic aneurysm (AAA)?

Population studied

Consecutive patients undergoing elective surgery for AAA between 1977 and 1988 were included. Only eight patients with some missing data were excluded. The mean age was 68 years.

Study size

The rule was developed using data from patients in 15 previous studies; it was then evaluated in 238 patients.

Pretest probability

The overall mortality rate was 5%.

Type of validation

Grade I/IV: The training group was used as the validation group, although literature data were originally used to develop the rule, which was then adjusted for the local pretest probability.

Comments

This rule is unusual in that it explicitly takes into account the mortality at a particular center in the rule itself. The definitions are clear. The validation technique is not simply "training group used as validation group"; the authors used data from the literature, calculated odds ratios, and then adjusted them specifically for their population. Thus the validation technique is better than a simple "training group used as validation group" would indicate.

Reference

Steyerberg EW, Kievit J, de Mol Van Otterloo JC, et al. Perioperative mortality of elective abdominal aortic aneurysm surgery. Arch Intern Med 1995;155:1998–2004.

CLINICAL PREDICTION RULE

1. Find your hospital or medical center's average surgical mortality.

Mortality	Points
3%	−5
4%	−2
5%	0
6%	+2
8%	+5
12%	+10

2. Add up your patient's individual prognostic factors:

Factor	Score
Age (years)	
60	−4
70	0
80	+4
Gender	
Male	
Female	+4
Cardiac co-morbidity[a]	
MI	+3
CHP	+8
ECG ischemia	+8
Serum creatinine (mg/dl)	
<1.8	0
≥1.8	+12
Pulmonary co-morbidity[b]	
Impaired	+7
Total:	

[a]MI = documented history of MI; CHF = cardiogenic pulmonary edema and/or jugular versus distension, or the presence of a gallop rhythm regardless of treatment; ECG ischemia: ST segment depression > 2 mm on a standard resting ECG.

[b]Pulmonary co-morbidity: chronic obstructive pulmonary disease (COPD), emphysema, or dyspnea, or had undergone previous pulmonary surgery.

3. Find total score from 1 and 2 above:

Total score	Mortality
−5	1%
0	2%
5	3%
10	5%
15	8%
20	12%
25	19%
30	28%
35	39%
40	51%

■ VENOUS THROMBOEMBOLISM (DEEP VEIN THROMBOSIS AND PULMONARY EMBOLISM)

Diagnosis of Deep Vein Thrombosis

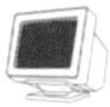

Clinical question

Which patients with suspected deep vein thrombosis (DVT) actually have one?

Population and setting

Outpatients referred for the evaluation of suspected DVT to a tertiary care hospital thrombosis clinic were included. They were excluded if pregnant, had had a lower extremity amputation or suspected PE, had symptoms for more than 60 days, or were currently using anticoagulants. The mean age was 57.1 years; 40% were male.

Study size

Altogether, 593 patients were studied.

Pretest probability

A DVT was diagnosed in 16%.

Type of validation

Grade I: The validation group was from a distinct population. The rule was developed in one group of patients and validated in another.

Comments

This is a well validated and useful clinical rule. It helps you accurately estimate the pretest probability of DVT, which in turn guides both your selection and interpretation of further tests.

References

Wells P, Anderson DR, Bormanis J, et al. Value of assessment of pretest probability of deep-vein thrombosis in clinical management. Lancet 1997;350:1795–1798.

Wells PS, Hirsh J, Anderson DR, Lensing AW, et al. Accuracy of clinical assessment of deep-vein thrombosis. Lancet 1995;345:1326–1330.

CLINICAL PREDICTION RULE

1. Count the number of risk factors for your patient and calculate their risk score.

Risk factor	Points
Active cancer (treatment ongoing or within previous 6 months or palliative)	1
Paralysis, paresis, or recent plaster immobilization of the lower extremities	1
Recently bedridden for >3 days of major surgery within 4 weeks	1
Localized tenderness along the distribution of the deep venous system	1
Entire leg swelling	1
Calf swelling by >3 cm when compared with the asymptomatic leg (measured 10 cm below the tibial tuberosity)	1
Pitting edema (greater in the symptomatic leg)	1
Collateral superficial veins (nonvaricose)	1
Alternative diagnosis as likely as or greater than that of DVT	−2
Total:	

2. Determine their pretest likelihood of DVT.

Risk score	Risk category	Probability of DVT (95% CI)
≤0	Low	3.0% (1.7%–5.9%)
1–2	Moderate	16.6% (12%–23%)
≥3	High	74.6% (63%–84%)

3. Based on your patients risk category, pursue the rest of the workup for DVT. USN = ultrasonography.

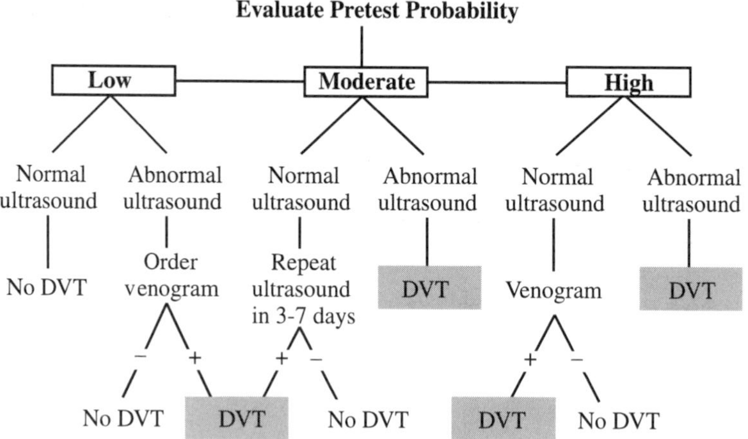

Risk of Thromboembolism in Patients with Nonvalvular Atrial Fibrillation

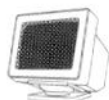

Clinical question

What is the risk of thromboembolism (pulmonary embolism or deep vein thrombosis) in patients with nonvalvular atrial fibrillation (NVAF)?

Population and setting

Data came from the placebo arm of the Stroke Prevention in Atrial Fibrillation (SPAF) trial, a large multicenter study comparing warfarin, aspirin, and placebo. Patients with nonvalvular atrial fibrillation were followed for a mean of 1.3 years.

Study size

Altogether, 568 patients were studied.

Pretest probability

Venous thromboembolism was seen in 6.3% during the follow-up period.

Type of validation

Grade IV: The training group and validation group were the same patients.

Comments

This rule is limited by the absence of prospective validation and should be used with caution. However, given the current standard of care (i.e., aspirin or warfarin for patients with NVAF, depending on their risk factors) it is unlikely that this type of study will be repeated prospectively.

Reference

SPAF Investigators. Predictors of thromboembolism in atrial fibrillation. I. Clinical features of patients at risk. Ann Intern Med 1992;116:1–5.

CLINICAL PREDICTION RULE

1. Count your patient's risk factors:

Risk factor	Points
History of hypertension	1
Recent congestive heart failure	1
Previous thromboembolism	1
Total:	

2. The patient's risk of thromboembolism is as follows.

Risk score	Risk of thromboembolism per year
0	2.5%
1	7.2%
2–3	17.6%

Diagnosis of Pulmonary Embolism I

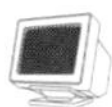

Clinical question

Which patients undergoing arteriography for suspected pulmonary embolism (PE) will have a positive test.

Population and setting

Adult patients undergoing pulmonary angiography for suspected PE at teaching hospitals in Omaha, Nebraska, were included. The median age was 59 years (range 14–84 years); 54% were male.

Study size

There were 101 patients in the training group and 68 in the validation group.

Pretest probability

Of the validation group, 28% had a positive arteriogram.

Type of validation

Grade II: The validation group was a separate sample from the same population, with data for the validation group gathered prospectively.

Comments

Although small, this rule was well designed and well validated. It does a good job of identifying patients at very low (score < 10) and very high (score > 19) risk of PE. There is a selection bias, as all patients had been scheduled for arteriography. It is unclear whether the rule would apply to a lower risk group of patients.

Reference

Hoellerich VL, Wigton RS. Diagnosing pulmonary embolism using clinical findings. Arch Intern Med 1986;146:1699–1704.

CLINICAL PREDICTION RULE

1. Add up the number of points for your patient.

Finding	Score
Age < 65	3
Diagnosis of cancer	4
Leg pain	3
Substernal chest pain	−3
Heart rate increase by > 20 beats/min	4
Heart rate > 90 beats/min	4
New S3 or S4	−4
Positive lung scan	5
Correction factor (add this to all scores)	8
Total:	

2. Use the table below to interpret the results.

Score	With pulmonary embolism
1–10	0%
11–18	38%
19–23	89%
24–31	100%

Diagnosis of Pulmonary Embolism II

Clinical question

Which patients with suspected pulmonary embolism (PE) actually have one?

Population and setting

Consecutive adult patients referred for suspected PE and enrolled in a study of the accuracy of perfusion scans alone were included. The mean age was 68 years (range 15–91 years); 49% were male.

Study size

The training group had 500 patients and the validation group 250.

Pretest probability

The prevalence of PE was 40% in the training group and 42% in the validation group.

Type of validation

Grade II: The validation group was a separate sample from the same population, with data for the validation group gathered prospectively.

Comments

The reference standard was pulmonary angiography for all patients with an abnormal perfusion scan (anything other than a normal or near-normal scan). Approximately 80% therefore underwent angiography. This type of bias (called verification bias) can cause the accuracy of the algorithm to be overestimated. However, other studies such as PIOPED have shown that the risk of PE in patients with normal or near-normal scans is only 2–3%, so any inflation is likely small.

Reference

Miniati M, Prediletto R, Formichi B, et al. Accuracy of clinical assessment in the diagnosis of pulmonary embolism. Am J Respir Crit Care Med 1999;159:864–871.

CLINICAL PREDICTION RULE

1. Count the number of key symptoms associated with pulmonary embolism.

   Sudden onset of dyspnea
   Chest pain
   Fainting

2. Determine whether your patient has a low, intermediate, or high risk of PE.

   High probability of PE (90%): Presence of at least one of the above three key symptoms *and* any two of the following abnormalities: (1) ECG signs of right ventricular overload; (2) radiographic signs of oligemia*; (3) amputation of the hilar artery†; or (4) pulmonary consolidations compatible with infarction.

   Intermediate probability of PE (50%): Presence of at least one of the above three key symptoms but not associated with the above electrocardiographic (ECG) and radiographic abnormalities, or associated with ECG signs of right ventricular overload only.‡

   Low probability of PE (10%): Absence of the above three key symptoms or identification of an alternative diagnosis that may account for their presence (e.g., exacerbation of COPD, pneumonia, lung edema, myocardial infarction, pneumothorax, and others).

*Oligemia was considered to be present if, in a given lung region, the pulmonary vasculature was greatly diminished with concomitant hyperlucency of the lung parenchyma.

†Amputation of the hilar artery gives the hilum a "plump" appearance.

‡ECG signs of right ventricular overload: S1Q3 pattern (with or without T wave inversion in lead III), S1S2S3 pattern, T wave inversion in right precordial leads, transient right bundle branch block (RBBB), and pseudoinfarction.

Risk of Bleeding Among Patients on an Anticoagulant

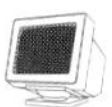

Clinical question

Which patients being treated with an anticoagulant for venous thromboembolism are at risk for bleeding complications?

Population and setting

The study population consisted of 1021 consecutive patients with objectively confirmed venous thromboembolism (deep vein thrombosis or pulmonary embolism). Half initially received low-molecular-weight heparin, and half received continuous unfractionated heparin; then all received warfarin for at least 3 months with an INR goal of 2.0–3.0. The mean age was 60 years in the validation group; 51% were male.

Study size

The validation group had 241 patients, and the validation set had 780 patients.

Pretest probability

Of 780 patients, 71 (9.1%) had a bleeding complication. Of these, 19 were considered major (clinically overt and a decline in hemoglobin concentration of at least 20 g/L, a need for transfusion of 2 units or more, located retroperitoneally or intracranially, or warranted permanent discontinuation of treatment).

Type of Validation

Grade I: The validation group was from a distinct population. The rule was developed in one group of patients and validated in another. The score was developed from the literature; cutpoints were identified; and the score was simplified using the validation group and validated in the validation set.

Comments

This thoughtfully designed and carefully validated rule is easy to apply. Patients should be monitored more carefully for bleeding complications in the high than those at low risk.

Reference

Kuijer PM, Hutten BA, Prins MH, Buller HR. Prediction of the risk of bleeding during anticoagulant treatment for venous thromboembolism. Arch Intern Med 1999; 159:457–460.

CLINICAL PREDICTION RULE

1. Add up your patient's risk score.

Risk factor	Points
Age ≥ 60 years	1.6
Female gender	1.3
Malignancy present	2.2
Total:	

2. Find the risk of bleeding complications in the table below.

No. of points	No. of patients in this group	No. with any bleeding complication	No. with major bleeding complication
0	170	6 (4%)	1 (1%)
1–3	460	39 (8%)	8 (2%)
>3	150	26 (17%)	10 (7%)

■ CONGESTIVE HEART FAILURE

ICU Prognosis for Patients with Congestive Heart Failure

Clinical question

What is the risk for in-hospital death for intensive care unit (ICU) patients with congestive heart failure (CHF)?

Population studied

All patients with a clinical diagnosis of CHF from their attending physician who were admitted to the ICU were included. Patients were excluded if it was the second admission for the same patient. If two patients were admitted simultaneously, the study nurse randomly selected one for study inclusion and data gathering. The study was set at a university hospital between 1982 and 1985. Patients had a mean age of 69 years (range 35–95 years); 46% were male.

Study size

The same 191 patients made up the training and validation groups (see type of validation below).

Pretest probability

The in-hospital mortality rate was 8.9%.

Type of validation

Grade III: This was a jackknife validation process: a fraction of the population was used as the validation group and the remainder as the training group; this was repeated until all patients had been part of the validation group.

Comments

Jackknife validation is a type of split-sample validation, where a fraction of the patient population (perhaps 10%) is pulled from the overall group and used as a validation group; then the process is repeated until each patient has served in a validation group. This is the statistical equivalent of split-sample validation, with the advantage of having a larger training group. This rule should be used with caution because of the vagueness of some of the predictor variable definitions ("diagnosis of congestive heart failure by attending physician," "clinical response during first 24 hours"). On the other hand, this is potentially more broadly generalizable than a rule with multiple inclusion and exclusion criteria.

Reference

Esdaile JM, Horwitz RI, Levinton C, et al. Response to initial therapy and new onset as predictors of prognosis in patients hospitalized with congestive heart failure. Clin Invest Med 1992;15:122–131.

CLINICAL PREDICTION RULE

1. Add up the points for your patient.

Variable	Points
Age ≥ 70 years	1
Presence of chest pain	1
Jugulovenous distension (JVD)	1
Level 2 or 3 of a cardiac severity scale (severe or life-threatening ischemia, arrhythmia, or valvular disease)	1
First episode of CHF	1
Deterioration or no change in 24-hour response to therapy	1
Total:	

2. Determine your patient's mortality and duration of hospital and ICU stay.

Score	No. in category	ICU days (mean)	Hospital days (mean)	Mortality
0–1	40	3.3	9.3	0%
2	58	3.9	12.7	3.5%
3	54	5.2	14.7	7.4%
4	26	—	—	19.2%
≥5	7	—	—	85.7%
≥4	—	8.8	17.6	—

Prognosis in Dilated Cardiomyopathy

Clinical question

What is the prognosis for patients with severe dilated cardiomyopathy?

Population and setting

In this Japanese study, patients with dilated cardiomyopathy admitted to The Heart Institute of Japan between 1967 and 1985 were studied. The training group had 91 males and 20 females, with a mean age of 40 years. The validation group consisted of 35 males and 6 females with a mean age of 42 years. The patients were followed up for a mean of 51 months (range 3 months to 15 years). Patients received digitalis (148 patients), diuretics ($n = 150$), vasodilators ($n = 86$), and antiarrhythmic drugs ($n = 84$). Because of the age of the study, they did not receive angiotensin-converting enzyme (ACE) inhibitors.

Study size

The training group had 111 patients and the validation group 41.

Pretest probability

Of 152 patients, 70 (46%) died of cardiac causes during the follow-up.

Type of validation

Grade II: The test set was a separate sample from the same population, with data for the test set gathered prospectively.

Comments

The major limitation of this study is a lack of clarity for some of the definitions (i.e., high grade ventricular arrhythmia) and the age of the dataset. The number of premature ventricular beats (PVBs) observed on a 24-hour Holter monitor was also a useful predictor in the validation group: All patients with fewer than 2000 PVBs in 24 hours survived during the follow-up period, whereas 13 of 16 with more than 2000 PVBs did not survive.

Reference

Ogasawara S, Sekiguchi M, Hiroe M, et al. Prognosis of dilated cardiomyopathy: from a retrospective to a prospective study employing multivariate analysis. Jpn Circ J 1987;51:699–706.

CLINICAL PREDICTION RULE

1. Add up the scores on axis 1 and axis 2 for your patient.

Variable	Score
Axis 1	
Supraventricular arrhythmia	
No	−0.09
Yes	+0.14
Prolongation of QRS interval	
No	−0.18
Yes	+0.29
Low voltage	
No	−0.06
Yes	+0.48
Left axis deviation	
No	−0.06
Yes	+0.22
High grade ventricular arrhythmia based on 24-hour Holter	
No	−0.05
Yes	+0.11
NYHA functional classification	
I or II	−0.19
III	+0.21
IV	+0.41
Cardiothoracic ratio	
$< 55\%$	−0.26
55–64%	−0.01
$\geq 65\%$	+0.39
Left ventricular end diastolic pressure (mmHg)	
< 18	−0.16
≥ 18	+0.17
Election fraction	
$< 27\%$	+0.19
$\geq 27\%$	−0.17
Axis 1 score:	
Axis 2	
Supraventricular arrhythmia	
No	−0.19
Yes	+0.29
Low voltage	
No	−0.02
Yes	+0.18
Left axis deviation	
No	+0.12
Yes	−0.47
High grade ventricular arrhythmia based on 24-hour Holter	
No	+0.11
Yes	−0.23
NYHA functional classification	
I or II	−0.07
III	+0.98
IV	−0.54
Cardiothoracic ratio	
$< 55\%$	−0.41
55–64%	+0.62
$\geq 65\%$	−0.53
Axis 2 score:	

2. Interpretation, based on the 41 patients in the validation group, is as follows. Overall, 25/41 (61%) survived.

Axis 1	Axis 2	Survivors/total
Positive	Positive	2/2 (100%)
Positive	Negative	4/19 (21%)
Negative	Positive	7/7 (100%)
Negative	Negative	12/13 (92%)

A negative axis 1 score is an indicator of good prognosis. A positive axis 1 score and a negative axis 2 score are indicators of poor prognosis.

Left Ventricular Ejection Fraction after MI

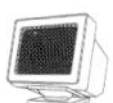

Clinical question

Which patients will have a normal left ventricular ejection fraction (LVEF) 2–21 days after myocardial infarction?

Population and setting

Consecutive patients at Massachusetts General Hospital with acute myocardial infarction (MI) were included. Those without a test for LVEF (17% of the total screened, a group that tended to have small infarcts) and a few who died early in the course of hospitalization (who probably had large infarcts) were excluded. Most patients (55%) were over age 65, and 69% were male. In the validation study of Krumholz et al., 1891 patients at community hospitals in Connecticut were studied (all over age 65; about 60% male). In Tobin et al.'s validation study, 213 patients were studied in a retrospective chart review at a community teaching hospital in Michigan.

Study size

In the original study, there were 162 patients in the training group and 152 in the validation group. Krumholz et al. studied 1891 patients, and Tobin et al. studied 213 in their validation studies.

Pretest probability

A normal LVEF was found in 45.3% of patients in the original study.

Type of validation

Grade II: The validation group was a separate sample from the same population, with data for the validation group gathered prospectively.

Comments

This simple rule divides patients into two groups: high risk and low risk. The prospective validations show that the rule does accurately identify a group of low risk patients, although the studies of Tobin et al. and Krumholz et al. showed that this group is not quite as low risk as found by Silver et al.

References

Krumholz HM, Howes CJ, Murillo JE, et al. Validation of a clinical prediction rule for left ventricular ejection fraction after myocardial infarction in patients ≥ 65 years old. Am J Cardiol 1997;80:11–15.

Silver MT, Rose GA, Paul SD, et al. A clinical rule to predict preserved left ventricular ejection fraction in patients after myocardial infarction. Ann Intern Med 1994;121:750–756.

Tobin K, Stomel R, Harber D, et al. Validation in a community hospital setting of a clinical rule to predict preserved left ventricular ejection fraction in patients after myocardial infarction. Arch Intern Med 1999;159:353–357.

CLINICAL PREDICTION RULE

1. Answer the following four questions yes or no about your patients.

Is there a history of congestive heart failure (CHF) or CHF with index MI?	Yes	No
Is the ECG uninterpretable [left bundle brash block (LBBB), pacing, left ventricular hypertrophy (LVH) with strain]?	Yes	No
Is there an old Q wave or Q wave outside the region of ischemia?	Yes	No
Is the MI anterior with new Q waves or ST elevations?	Yes	No

A patient is at "high risk for LVEF < 40%" if any of the above answers is "yes."

2. The results of the original study and two additional prospective validation studies are shown below.

Risk	Original study (n = 152)	Tobin et al. (n = 213)	Krumholz et al. (n = 1891)
High risk (yes to any question)	83 (43%)[a]	—	1378 (44%)
Low risk (no to all 4 questions)	69 (2%)	83 (14%)	513 (11%)

[a]Numbers in parentheses are the percent of patients with LVEF < 40%.

PREOPERATIVE EVALUATION

Goldman's Cardiac Risk Index

Clinical question

What is the risk of cardiac death and cardiac complications for patients undergoing noncardiac surgery?

Population and setting

In the original study of Goldman et al., consecutive patients over age 40 presenting to Massachusetts General Hospital for noncardiac surgery during the 1970s were included; patients with angina were excluded. Detsky et al. studied consecutive patients over age 40 presenting for noncardiac surgery at Toronto General Hospital during the 1980s; they did not exclude those with angina.

Study size

Altogether, 1001 patients were studied by Goldman et al. (used to derive the rule) and 455 in the study of Detsky et al.

Pretest probability

In the Goldman study 6% of patients had a cardiac complication of perioperative death, compared with 10% in the Detsky study.

Type of validation

Goldman, et al.—Grade IV: The training group was used as the validation group.
Detsky et al.—Grade I: The validation group was from a distinct population. The rule was developed in one group of patients and validated in another.

Comments

Although widely used, this score was not prospectively validated in the original study. Detsky and colleagues did a prospective, blinded validation in a different population. Both results are presented below. The Detsky results are preferred owing to the stronger validation method.

References

Detsky AS, Abrams HB, McLaughlin JR, et al. Predicting cardiac complications in patients undergoing non-cardiac surgery. J Gen Intern Med 1986;1:211–219.

Goldman L, Caldera D, Nussbaum SR, et al. Multifactorial index of cardiac risk in non-cardiac surgical procedures. N Engl J Med 1977;197:845–850.

CLINICAL PREDICTION RULE

1. Add up the points for your patient.

Risk factor	Points
History of myocardial infarction (one only):	
Within the past 6 months	10
More than 6 months ago	5
Physical examination	
S3 or jugular venous distension	11
Important aortic stenosis	3
Electrocardiogram	
Rhythm other than sinus or sinus plus atrial premature beats	7
More than five premature ventricular beats per minute at any time preoperatively	7
Poor general medical status:	
any of the following: $PO_2 < 60$ mm Hg, $PCO_2 > 50$ mm Hg, $K^+ < 3.0$ mEq/L, $HCO_3 < 20$ mEq/L, BUN > 50 mg/dl, creatinine > 3 mg/dl, abnormal SGOT, signs of chronic liver disease, or bedridden from noncardiac causes	3
Intraperitoneal, intrathoracic, or aortic surgery	3
Age over 70 years	5
Emergency operation	4
Total (maximum 53):	

2. Find his or her risk of cardiac complications and death (data from Goldman et al.'s original study).

		Probability of cardiac complications	
Risk class	Likelihood ratio for cardiac complications	Pretest probability of 5%	Pretest Probability of 10%
I (0–5 points)	0.15	0.8%	1.6%
II (6–12 points)	1.2	5.9%	11.8%
III (13–25 points)	2.6	12.0%	22.4%
IV (>25 points)	60.0	75.9%	87.0%

3. Find his or her risk of cardiac complications below (data from prospective validation at Toronto General Hospital by Detsky and colleagues).

		Probability of cardiac complications	
Risk class	Likelihood ratio for cardiac complications	Pretest probability of 5%	Pretest probability of 10%
I (0–5 points)	0.56	2.9%	5.9%
II (6–12 points)	0.62	3.2%	6.4%
III (13–25 points)	2.25	10.6%	20.1%
IV (> 25 points)	Infinity[a]	84.0%	91.7%

[a]A likelihood ratio of 100 was used to calculate the probabilities of cardiac complications.

Detsky's Modified Cardiac Risk Index

Clinical question

What is the risk of cardiac death and cardiac complications for patients undergoing noncardiac surgery?

Population and setting

Consecutive patients over age 40 presenting at Toronto General Hospital for noncardiac surgery with "a question of cardiac risk" were included. Patients with angina were not excluded.

Study size

Altogether, 455 were studied.

Pretest probability

A cardiac complication was seen in 10% of patients.

Type of validation

Grade I: The validation group was from a distinct population. The rule was developed in one group of patients and validated in another.

Comments

This rule is a modification of Goldman's original rule. It is somewhat more accurate, includes patients with angina, and has been prospectively validated. A nomogram is included to simplify the application of this important rule to your local hospital conditions. The pretest probabilities in the nomogram are from Detsky et al.'s experience at Toronto General Hospital.

References

Detsky AS, Abrams HB, Forbath N, Scott JG, Hilliard JR. Cardiac assessment for patients undergoing noncardiac surgery: a multifactorial clinical risk index. Arch Intern Med 1986;146:2131–2134.

Detsky AS, Abrams HB, McLaughlin JR, et al. Predicting cardiac complications in patients undergoing non-cardiac surgery. J Gen Intern Med 1986;1:211–219.

CLINICAL PREDICTION RULE

1. Add up the points for your patient.

Risk factor	Points
Myocardial infarction (select one only)	
MI within 6 months	10
MI more than 6 months ago	5
Angina (select one only)	
Class III: angina occurring with level walking of one to two blocks or climbing one flight of stairs or less at a normal pace	10
Class IV: inability to carry on any physical activity without the development of angina	20
Unstable angina within 6 months[a]	10
Alveolar pulmonary edema (select one only)[b]	
Within 1 week	10
Ever	5
Suspected critical aortic stenosis[c]	20
Electrocardiogram (select all that apply)	
Rhythm other than sinus or sinus plus atrial premature beats on last preoperative ECG	5
More than five premature ventricular beats per minute at any time prior to surgery	5
Poor general medical status:	
any of the following: $PO_2 < 60$ mm Hg, $PCO_2 > 50$ mm Hg, $K^+ < 3.0$ mEq/L, $HCO_3 < 20$ mEq/L, BUN > 50 mg/dl, creatinine > 3 mg/dl, abnormal SGOT, signs of chronic liver disease, or bedridden from noncardiac causes	5
Age over 70 years	5
Emergency operation	10
Total (maximum 105):	

[a]Unstable angina was defined as new-onset angina (within 1 month) occurring with minimal exertion, an episode of coronary insufficiency, crescendo angina, or angina occurring at rest as well as with minimal exertion. Patients who had little or no angina with exertion but who had most of their angina occurring at rest in a stable pattern were diagnosed as having atypical angina and not considered unstable.

[b]Alveolar pulmonary edema within 1 week of surgery: physical signs (S3 gallop, respiratory distress, rales elevated jugular pressure) and chest radiograph findings of alveolar edema. Diagnosed "ever" if the patient had a history of severe respiratory distress relieved by diuretics and the patient was given a diagnosis consistent with pulmonary edema by a physician.

[c]Suspected critical aortic stenosis: suspicion of a 50 mm Hg gradient across the aortic valve based on history (syncope on exertion), physical examination (slow and low-volume carotid upstroke with vigorous left ventricular impulse), and left ventricular hypertrophy on ECG.

2a. *Major surgery.* Find the risk of cardiac complications (myocardial infarction, death, or congestive heart failure) for major surgery. Major surgery includes intraperitoneal, intrathoracic, retroperitoneal, aortic, carotid vascular, peripheral vascular, neurosurgical, major orthopedic, and major head and neck surgery.

		Probability of cardiac complications	
Risk class	Likelihood ratio for cardiac complications	Pretest probability of 5%	Pretest probability of 10%
I (0–15 points)	0.4	2.2%	4.5%
II (20–30 points)	3.6	15.9%	28.5%
III (> 30 points)	14.9	44.0%	62.3%

2b. *Minor surgery.* Find the risk of cardiac complications (myocardial infarction, death, or congestive heart failure) for minor surgery. Minor surgery includes transurethral resection of prostate, cataract surgery, minor head and neck surgery, and minor orthopedic procedures such as arthroscopy.

Risk class	Likelihood ratio for cardiac complications	Probability of cardiac complications	
		Pretest probability of 1%	Pretest probability of 3%
I (0–15 points)	0.4	0.4%	1.2%
II (20–30 points)	2.8	2.7%	7.8%
III (> 30 points)	12.2	11.0%	27.4%

3. For the most accurate possible estimate, take into account the pretest probability of a perioperative cardiac complication at your institution using the nomogram below. This nomogram can be used to calculate the risk of a perioperative cardiac complication. Find the patient's pretest probability of a complication for that procedure at your institution on the left-hand line. Draw a straight line through the patient's risk score on the center line, and find the probability of a perioperative cardiac complication in the right-hand line.

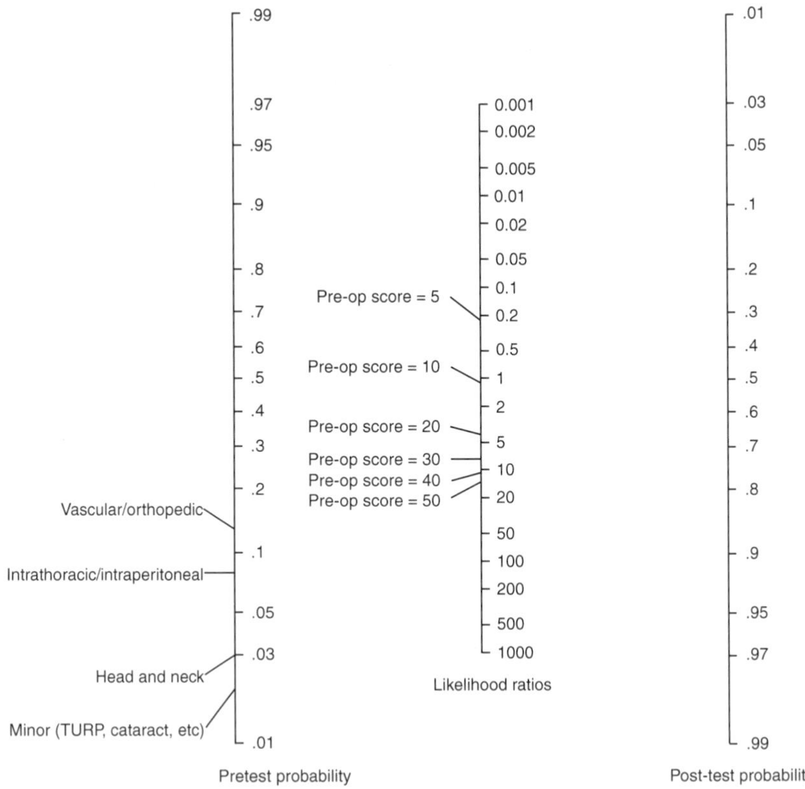

Cardiac Risk during Vascular Surgery

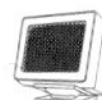

Clinical question

What is the risk of cardiac complications among patients undergoing vascular surgery?

Population and setting

Patients referred to Massachusetts General Hospital or the University of Massachusetts Medical Center for dipyridamole-thallium testing before major elective vascular surgery were included. Thirty-nine were excluded because their surgery was cancelled owing to severe coronary disease. Most were under age 70 (58.4%), 43.6% were male, and 56% had a history of a Q wave myocardial infarction (MI).

Study size

There were 567 patients in the training group and 514 in the validation group

Pretest probability

Of patients in the validation group, 7.6% had a major cardiac event (nonfatal MI or cardiac death).

Type of validation

Grade I: The validation group was from a distinct population. The rule was developed in one group of patients and validated in another.

Comments

This well validated clinical prediction rule predicts the likelihood of cardiac complications among patients referred for stress thallium tests prior to major elective vascular surgery. Thus it does not apply to patients undergoing emergent procedures or non-vascular surgery. It is actually two rules: the first for patients who have not had a stress thallium test and the second incorporating the results of that test if available. Also, the test takes into account a center's overall complication rate for vascular surgery, an important and appropriate adjustment. One limitation: diabetes mellitus is not defined.

Reference

L'Italien GJ, Paul SD, Hendel RC, et al. Development and validation of a bayesian model for perioperative cardiac risk assessment in a cohort of 1,081 vascular surgical candidates. J Am Coll Cardiol 1996;27:779–786.

CLINICAL PREDICTION RULE

1. First, calculate the clinical score.

Variable	Points
Age > 70	0.5
Diabetes	0.8
Angina	0.8
Congestive heart failure	0.6
Prior infarction	0.5
Prior bypass (within last 5 years)	−2.2
Clinical score:	

2. Then find the major perioperative cardiac event corresponding to your patient's clinical score and the complication rate at your institution.

	Complication rate at your institution							
Clinical score	2%	4%	6%	8%	10%	12%	14%	16%
0–	1%	2%	3%	4%	5%	6%	7%	8%
0.5	1%	2%	3%	4%	5%	6%	7%	8%
>0.5–	1%	3%	4%	6%	7%	9%	11%	12%
1.0	2%	3%	5%	7%	8%	10%	12%	13%
>1.0–	3%	5%	8%	10%	13%	15%	18%	20%
1.5	4%	8%	11%	15%	18%	21%	24%	27%
>1.5–	4%	8%	12%	16%	19%	23%	26%	29%
2.0	6%	12%	17%	22%	27%	31%	35%	38%
>2.0–	7%	13%	19%	24%	29%	33%	37%	41%
2.5	10%	18%	25%	32%	37%	42%	47%	50%
>2.5–	11%	20%	27%	34%	40%	45%	49%	53%
3.0	15%	27%	36%	43%	50%	55%	59%	63%

3. If your patient has had a dipyridamole stress thallium test, calculate his or her thallium risk score.

Variable	Points
Ischemic ST changes	
(≥1 mm ST segment depression)	1.2
Fixed defect	0.8
Reversible defect	1.3
Thallium risk score:	

4. Then find the percent risk of cardiac complications below corresponding to the thallium risk score and clinical risk above.

	Clinical risk from step 2 above							
Thallium risk score	2.5%	5.0%	7.5%	10.0%	12.5%	15.0%	17.5%	20.0%
0–	1%	1%	2%	2%	3%	4%	4%	5%
0.5	1%	1%	2%	3%	3%	4%	5%	6%
>0.5–	1%	2%	3%	4%	5%	6%	7%	8%
1.0	1%	2%	3%	4%	5%	7%	8%	9%
>1.0–	2%	3%	5%	7%	8%	10%	12%	14%
1.5	2%	5%	7%	10%	12%	15%	17%	20%
>1.5–	3%	5%	8%	11%	13%	16%	19%	21%
2.0	4%	7%	11%	15%	19%	22%	25%	29%
>2.0–	4%	8%	13%	16%	20%	24%	27%	31%
2.5	6%	12%	18%	23%	27%	32%	36%	40%
>2.5–	7%	13%	19%	24%	29%	34%	38%	42%
3.0	10%	18%	26%	33%	38%	43%	48%	52%
>3.0–	12%	21%	30%	37%	43%	48%	53%	57%
3.5	14%	24%	34%	42%	48%	53%	58%	62%

Morbidity and Mortality Following Cardiac Surgery

Clinical question

What is the risk of complications and death among patients undergoing cardiac surgery?

Population and setting

Consecutive adult patients undergoing cardiac surgery were included; patients undergoing ventricular aneurysmectomy, endocardial mapping, carotid endarterectomy, or nonvalvular intracardiac surgery were excluded. Only 3% represented emergency surgery. Regarding age, 35% were age 65–74 years, and approximately 16% were over age 74.

Study size

The training group had 3156 patients and the validation group 394.

Pretest probability

The overall complication rate was 22%, and the rate of death was 6.2%.

Type of validation

Grade II: The validation group was a separate sample from the same population, with data for the validation group gathered prospectively.

Comments

This large study used prospective data collection to create the prediction rule. It performed well in validation on a separate group of patients.

Reference

Tuman KJ, McCarthy RJ, March RJ, et al. Morbidity and duration of ICU stay after cardiac surgery: a model for preoperative risk assessment. Chest 1992;102:36–44.

CLINICAL PREDICTION RULE

1. Calculate the risk score for your patient.

Risk factor	Points
Emergency surgery	4
Age (years)	
65–74	1
>74	2
Renal dysfunction (creatinine >1.4 mg/dl)	2
Previous myocardial infarction (select one only)	
Between 3 and 6 months ago	1
Less than 3 months ago	2
Female gender	2
Reoperation	2
Pulmonary hypertension (mean pulmonary arterial pressure >25% of systemic values)	2
Cerebrovascular disease (preoperatively)	2
Congestive heart failure (typical chest radiograph with S3 or rales)	1
Left ventricular dysfunction (ejection fraction <0.35)	1
Type of surgery (select one only)	
Multivalve or CABG + valve surgery	2
Mitral or aortic valve surgery	1
Total:	

2. Find the risk of complications below (data from the validation group of 394 patients).

Risk category	No. of patients	Observed rate of complications
Low (0–5 points)	292	14.7%
Moderate (6–9 points)	85	30.6%
High (>9 points)	17	52.9%

3. Find the risk of specific types of complications and death. (*Note:* Data are from the training group of 3156 patients; hence the type of validation for these data is grade IV.) Values for risk of complications are expressed as a percentage.

Outcome	0–1	2–3	4–5	6–7	8–9	10–11	>11	Overall
No. of cases	433	949	823	483	277	135	56	3,156
% With ≥1 complications	5.8	14.3	20.0	30.4	39.7	55.6	75.0	22.2
% With >2 complications	1.2	3.4	5.9	10.2	19.1	28.9	46.4	8.1
% With renal insufficiency	0.5	1.4	4.7	8.1	10.1	13.3	25.0	4.8
% With CNS complications	0.2	1.8	2.7	5.4	7.9	11.1	19.6	3.6
% With serious infection	1.8	3.4	4.0	6.0	9.4	14.1	16.1	4.9
% Operative mortality	0.5	1.7	1.5	1.9	4.0	9.6	16.1	2.3
% Overall mortality	1.6	3.5	4.3	7.0	11.9	24.4	39.3	6.2
ICU stay in days (SD deviation)	2.2 ± 0.7	2.6 ± 1.7	3.3 ± 3.6	4.0 ± 5.8	5.4 ± 7.5	6.5 ± 9.0	8.2 ± 10.7	3.5 ± 4.5

3

Critical Care

MORTALITY PREDICTION

APACHE II Score

Clinical question

What is the prognosis for a patient in the intensive care unit (ICU)?

Population and setting

Consecutive patients admitted to the ICUs of 13 hospitals were included. Approximately half of the patients were postoperative, 1–11% (depending on the hospital) had cancer, and approximately 40% were over age 65.

Study size

Altogether, 5815 ICU patients at 13 hospitals were studied, of whom 5030 (86%) had all variables measured and therefore contributed to the study results.

Pretest probability

Of 5030 patients, 993 died (19.7%).

Type of validation

Grade I: The validation group was from a distinct population. The rule was developed in one group of patients and validated in another.

Comments

Like the Simplified Acute Physiology Score (SAPS) (see below), the variables and weights for the Acute Physiology and Chronic Health Evaluation (APACHE II) were chosen based on "clinical judgment and documented physiologic relationships." This score is widely used in American hospitals as a way to measure quality of care. For example, if patients with similar APACHE II scores have different mortality rates in two ICUs, it is appropriate to question why that is the case. Its validation is limited to the ICU setting.

References

Bosscha K, Reijders K, Hulstaert F, Algra A, van der Werken C. Prognostic scoring systems to predict outcome in peritonitis and intra-abdominal sepsis. Br J Surg 1997;84:1532–1534.

Knaus WA, Draper EA, Wagner DP, Zimmerman JE. APACHE II: a severity of disease classification system. Crit Care Med 1985;13:818–829.

CLINICAL PREDICTION RULE

1. Add up the acute physiology points for your patient. Use the most abnormal reading during the patient's initial 24 hours in the ICU. (See page 110 for table.)
2. Add up the *age* and *chronic health* points:

Age (years)	Points
<45	0
45–54	2
55–64	3
65–74	5
>74	6

Chronic health points: If the patient has a history of severe organ system insufficiency or is immune-compromised assign points as follows.

Nonoperative or emergency postoperative patients: 5 points
Elective postoperative patients: 2 points

Definitions
Organ insufficiency or immune-compromised state must have been evident prior to this hospital admission and conform to the following criteria.

Liver: biopsy-proven cirrhosis and documented portal hypertension; episodes of past upper gastrointestinal (GI) bleeding attributed to portal hypertension; or prior episodes of hepatic failure/encephalopathy/coma.

Cardiovascular: New York Heart Association (NYHA) class IV.

Respiratory: chronic restrictive, obstructive, or vascular disease resulting in severe exercise restriction (i.e., unable to climb stairs or perform household duties); or documented chronic hypoxia, hypercapnia, secondary polycythemia, severe pulmonary hypertension (>40 mm Hg) or respirator dependence.

Renal: Receiving chronic dialysis.

Immune-compromised: The patient has received therapy that suppresses resistance to infection (e.g., immune suppression, chemotherapy, irradiation, long-term or recent high-dose steroids) or has a disease that is sufficiently advanced to suppress resistance to infection (e.g., leukemia, lymphoma, AIDS).

3. The total APACHE II score is the sum of a, b, and c:
   a. Acute Physiology Score ________________
   b. Age points ________________
   c. Chronic health points ________________
   Total APACHE II score: ________________
4. Interpret the APACHE II score: Find the APACHE II score in the left-hand column and the risk of in-hospital death in the appropriate column to the right. Note that the APACHE II should not be used for individual patient decision-making but is appropriate for health system and ICU comparisons. Percentages were taken from figures, and may be off by 1–2%.

Parameter	Points assigned 4	3	2	1	0	1	2	3	4	Points
Temperature (rectal) (°C)	≥41	39–40.9		38.5–38.9	36–38.4	34–35.9	32–33.9	30–31.9	≤29.9	
Mean arterial pressure (mm Hg)	≥160	130–159	110–129		70–109		50–69		≤49	
Heart rate (ventricular resp.)	≥180	140–179	110–139		70–109		55–69	40–54	≤39	
Respiratory rate (nonventilated or ventilated)	≥50	35–49		25–34	12–24	10–11	6–9		≤5	
Oxygenation	≥500	350–499	200–349		<200					
$FiO_2 \geq 0.5$: record A-aDO_2										
$FiO_2 < 0.5$: record only PaO_2					$PO_2 > 70$	PO_2 61–70		PO_2 55–60	$PO_2 < 55$	
Arterial pH	≥7.7	7.60–7.69		7.50–7.59	7.33–7.49		7.25–7.32	7.15–7.24	<7.15	
Serum sodium (mmol/L)	≥180	160–179	155–159	150–154	130–149		120–129	111–119	≤110	
Serum potassium (mmol/L)	≥7.0	6.0–6.9		5.5–5.9	3.5–5.4	3.0–3.4	2.5–2.9		<2.5	
Serum creatinine (mg/dl)[a]	≥3.5	2.0–3.4	1.5–1.9		0.6–1.4		<0.6			
Hematocrit (%)	≥60		50.0–59.9	46.0–49.9	30.0–45.9		20.0–29.9		<20	
White blood cell count (1000/mm³)	≥40		20.0–39.9	15.0–19.9	3.0–14.9		1.0–2.9		<1	
Glasgow Coma Score (GCS)										
(=15 − actual GCS)										
Total acute physiology score										
Serum HCO_3 (venous) (mmol/L)[b]	≥52	41.0–51.9		32.0–40.9	22.0–31.9		18.0–21.9	15.0–17.9	<15	

[a]Double point score for *acute* renal failure.
[b]Not preferred, use if no arterial blood gas done.

	Hospital mortality					
APACHE score	Nonoperative patients	Postoperative patients	GI bleeding	Congestive health failure	Respiratory failure from infection	Septic shock
0–4	4%	1%	11%	0%	18%	28%
5–9	7%	3%				
10–14	14%	7%	27%	13%	23%	
15–19	24%	13%				
20–24	42%	29%	50%	45%	45%	55%
25–29	53%	35%				
30–34	71%	71%	77%	75%	88%	80%
>34	83%	88%				

For patients with peritonitis and intraabdominal sepsis, a small independent validation in a Dutch hospital found the following.

APACHE II score	Deaths/total patients with that score
0–19	7/34 (21%)
≥20	15/16 (94%)

Simplified Acute Physiology Score

Clinical question

What is the prognosis for a patient in the intensive care unit (ICU)?

Population and setting

The Simplified Acute Physiology Score (SAPS) was evaluated in 679 unselected patients from eight ICUs. All data were collected during the first 24 hours after admission. There was no detailed information given about demographics, although 40% had undergone surgery, and 30% were hospital transfers.

Study size

The validation group had 679 patients.

Pretest probability

The overall mortality rate was 27.2%.

Type of validation

Grade I: The validation group was from a distinct population. The rule was developed in one group of patients and validated in another.

Comments

The authors do not give many details on how they developed this rule, although in this study it was prospectively validated. We also do not know much about the demographics of the included patients. For these reasons and the fact that the SAPS was validated in French patients, the APACHE II is the preferred acute physiology score, at least in the United States.

References

Bosscha K, Reijders K, Hulstaert F, Algra A, van der Werken C. Prognostic scoring systems to predict outcome in peritonitis and intra-abdominal sepsis. Br J Surg 1997;84:1532–1534.

Le Gall J-R, Loirat P, Alperovitch A, et al. A simplified acute physiology score for ICU patients. Crit Care Med 1984;12:975–979.

CLINICAL PREDICTION RULE

1. Add up the points for your patient. (See page 114 for table.)
2. The ICU mortality rate is shown below.

SAPS	No. of patients	Mortality rate (SD)
4	64	—
5–6	56	10.7% (4.1)
7–8	75	13.3% (3.9)
9–10	103	19.4% (7.8)
11–12	106	24.5% (4.1)
13–14	70	30.0% (5.5)
15–16	81	32.1% (5.1)
17–18	43	44.2% (7.6)
19–20	28	50.0% (9.4)
>20	53	81.1% (5.4)

3. For patients with peritonitis and intraabdominal sepsis, a small independent validation in a Dutch hospital found the following.

SAPS	Deaths/total patients with that score
0–19	8/34 (23%)
≥20	14/16 (88%)

Parameter	Points assigned 4	3	2	1	0	1	2	3	4	Points
Age (years)					≤ 45	46–55	56–65	66–75	> 75	
Heart rate (beats/min)	≥ 180	140–179	110–139		70–109		55–69	40–54	< 40	
Systolic BP (mm Hg)	≥ 190		150–189		80–149		55–79		< 55	
Body temperature (°C)	≥ 41	39.0–40.9		38.5–38.9	36.0–38.4	34.0–35.9	32.0–33.9	30.0–31.9	< 30.0	
Spontaneous resp. rate (if not on ventilator)	≥ 50	35–49		25–34	12–24	10–11	6–9		< 6	
Ventilator of CPAP								Yes		
Urinary output (L/24 hr)			>5.00	3.50–4.99	0.70–3.49		0.50–0.69	0.20–0.49	< 0.20	
BUN (mmol/L)	≥ 55.0	36.0–54.9	29.0–35.9	7.5–28.9	3.5–7.4	< 3.5				
Hematocrit (%)	≥ 60.0		50.0–59.9	46.0–49.9	30.0–45.9		20.0–29.9		< 20.0	
White blood cell count (1000/mm^3)	≥ 40.0		20.0–39.9	15.0–19.9	3.0–14.9		1.0–2.9		< 1.0	
Serum glucose (mmol/L)	≥ 44.5	27.8–44.4		14.0–27.7	3.9–13.9		2.8–3.8	1.6–2.7	< 1.6	
Serum potassium (mEq/L)	≥ 7.0	6.0–6.9		5.5–5.9	3.5–5.4	3.0–3.4	2.5–2.9		< 2.5	
Serum sodium (mEq/L)	≥ 180	161–179	156–160	151–155	130–150		130–120	110–119	< 110	
Serum HCO_3 (mEq/L)		> 40.0		30.0–39.9	20.0–29.9	10.0–19.9		5.0–9.9	< 5.0	
Glasgow Coma Score					13–15	10–12	7–9	4–6	3	
									Total:	

Simplified Acute Physiology Score II (SAPS II)

Clinical question

What is the risk of death for a patient in the intensive care unit (ICU)?

Population and setting

This was a large multicenter study in Europe and North America. All patients were hospitalized in the ICU, with a mean ICU length of stay of 6.6 days and a mean hospital length of stay of 19.1 days. The mean age was 57.2 years; 59.6% were male; and about half were surgical admissions (62% scheduled, 38% unscheduled).

Study size

The training group had 8549 patients and the validation group 4603.

Pretest probability

The overall mortality rate was 21.8%.

Type of validation

Grade II: The test set was a separate sample from the same population, with data for the test set gathered prospectively.

Comments

This is an updated version of the Simplified Acute Physiology Score. It was prospectively validated in a large population. Estimates of mortality should be used to compare ICUs, not to make individual care decisions.

Reference

LeGall J-R, Lemeshow S, Saulnier F. A new Simplified Acute Physiology Score (SAPS II) based on a European/NorthAmerican multicenter study. JAMA 1993;270:2957–2963.

CLINICAL PREDICITON RULE

1. Add up the number of points for your patient.

Variable	Points
Age (years)	
<40	0
40–59	7
60–69	12
70–74	15
75–79	16
≥80	18
Heart rate (beats/min, worst value in the first 24 hr)	
<40	11
40–69	2
70–119	0
120–159	4
≥160	7
Systolic BP (mm Hg, worst value in the first 24 hr)	
<70	13
70–99	5
100–199	0
≥200	2
Highest body temperature	
<39°C (102.2°F)	0
≥39°C (≥ 102.2°F)	3
Ratio of mm Hg/PaO_2 (only if ventilator or continuous pulmonary artery pressure; use lowest ratio)	
<100	11
100–199	9
≥200	6
Urinary output (liters/24 hr)[a]	
<0.5	11
0.5–0.999	4
≥1.0	0
Serum urea nitrogen (mg/dl; highest value)	
<28	0
28–83	6
≥84	10
White blood cell count (1000/mm^3; worst value)	
<1.0	12
1.0–19.9	0
≥20.0	3
Serum potassium (mmol/L; worst value)	
3.0–4.9	0
≥5.0	3
Serum sodium (mEq/L; worst value)	
<125	5
125–144	0
≥145	1
Serum HCO_3 (mEq/l; lowest value)	
<15	6
15–19	3
≥20	0
Serum bilirubin (mg/dl; highest value)	
<4.0	0
4.0–5.9	4
≥6.0	9

Variable	Points
Glasgow Coma Score (lowest value; if sedated, use value before sedation)	
<6	26
6–8	13
9–10	7
11–13	5
14–15	0
Chronic diseases[b]	
Metastatic cancer	9
Hematologic malignancy	10
AIDS	17
Type of admission[c]	
Scheduled surgical	0
Medical	6
Unscheduled surgical	8
Total:	

[a]Urinary output: If patient is in ICU less than 24 hours, adjust measurement to estimate full 24-hour value. For example, if it is 700 ml in 8 hours, enter 2100 ml for 24 hours.

[b]Metastatic cancer: confirmed by surgery, computed tomography, or any other method. Hematologic malignancy; yes, if lymphoma, multiple myeloma, or acute leukemia. AIDS: Yes, if HIV-positive with clinical complications such as *Pneumocystis carinii* pneumonia, Kaposi's sarcoma, lymphoma, tuberculosis or Toxoplasma.

[c]Scheduled surgical: surgery scheduled at least 24 hours in advance.

2. Find the patient's risk of death.

Score	Mortality
0	0%
5	0.4%
10	1.0%
15	2.0%
20	3.7%
22	4.7%
25	6.5%
27	7.9%
30	10.6%
32	12.8%
35	16.7%
37	19.6%
40	24.7%
42	28.5%
45	34.8%
47	39.2%
50	46.1%
55	57.5%
60	68.1%
65	76.9%
70	83.8%
75	88.9%
80	92.5%
85	95.0%
90	96.7%
95	97.8%
100	98.5%
>100	>98.5%

Mortality and Length of Stay after Cardiac Surgery

Clinical question

What is the risk of death and average length of stay for patients after cardiac surgery?

Population and setting

All adult patients undergoing cardiac surgery in Ontario during 1991 (training group) and 1992 (validation group) were included: 56% were under age 65 and 9% were 75 or older; 74% were male; 77% underwent CABG; and surgery was urgent or emergent in 34%.

Study size

The training group had 6213 patients and the validation group 6885 patients.

Pretest probability

The overall mortality rate was 3.7%, and the mean length of stay in the intensive care unit (ICU) was 3.2 days.

Type of validation

Grade II: The test set was a separate sample from the same population, with data for the test set gathered prospectively.

Comments

This is a large, prospective validation that is also easier to apply than some of the more general ICU risk models such as the SAPS or APACHE. As with any of these tools, it should not generally be used to influence individual patient decisions; rather, it provides prognostic information for a group of similar patients. It is useful for comparing ICUs and determining staffing needs.

Reference

Tu JV, Jagial SB, Naylo CD, et al. Multicenter validation of a risk index for mortality intensive care unit stay, and overall hospital length of stay after cardiac surgery. Circulation 1995;91:677–684.

CLINICAL PREDICTION RULE

Variable	Points
Age (years)	
<65	0
65–74	2
≥75	3
Gender	
Male	0
Female	1
Left ventricular function	
Grade 1 (EF > 50%)	0
Grade 2 (EF 35%–50%)	1
Grade 3 (EF 20%–34%)	2
Grade 4 (EF < 20%)	3
Type of surgery	
CABG only	0
Single valve	2
Complex (multivalve or CABG + valve)	3
Urgency of surgery	
Elective	0
Urgent	1
Emergent	4
Repeat operation	
No	0
Yes	2
Total (range 0–16):	

2. Determine the patient's predicted length of stay (LOS) and in-hospital mortality.

Risk score	Patients with this score (%)	In-hospital mortality rate	Mean ICU LOS (days)	Mean postoperative LOS (days)
0	11.8%	0.25%	2.3	8.0
1	14.7%	0.8%	2.4	8.4
2	17.8%	1.3%	2.8	9.3
3	17.1%	2.9%	2.9	10.4
4	14.2%	4.6%	3.2	11.0
5	10.7%	5.7%	3.3	11.4
6	6.4%	8.1%	3.7	12.8
7	3.9%	11.6%	4.3	13.1
≥8	3.3%	13.2%	5.9	14.5

Mortality Prediction Model

Clinical question

Which patients in the intensive care unit (ICU) survive to hospital discharge?

Population and setting

Consecutive patients admitted to the ICU at a regional medical center and teaching hospital were included. Patients were excluded if they had missing records (n = 12).

Study size

The training and validation group (same patients) included 755 patients.

Pretest probability

The overall mortality rate was 19.7%.

Type of validation

Grade IV: The training group was used as the validation group.

Comments

This rule has several limitations, most importantly the lack of independent validation, and it should be used with caution. The SAPS and APACHE II scores have both been better validated. Also, some of the predictor variables have the potential for ambiguity, such as "type of admission" and "number of organ system failures." The advantage of this score is mostly a theoretic one: that the variable weights were decided based on a logistic model rather than expert opinion.

Reference

Lemeshow S, Teres D, Pastides H, Avrunin JS, Steingrub JS. A method for predicting survival and mortality of ICU patients using objectively derived weights. Crit Care Med 1985;13:519–525.

CLINICAL PREDICTION RULE

1. Review the following definitions.

Coma: unresponsive to painful stimulation.

Deep stupor: minimal response to pain with decorticate or decerebrate posturing.

Emergency admission: medical patients admitted on an emergency basis plus emergency or urgent surgical cases.

Cancer: confirmed by operative pathology report, biopsy report, physician's operative note, and/or ICU admission note.

Confirmed infection: confirmed by culture, Gram stain, radiography, or presence of gross purulence.

Organ system failure: organ systems are cardiac, vascular, respiratory, gastrointestinal (including esophagus, liver, pancreas, gallbladder), neurologic, renal (including genitourinary), metabolic, and hematologic.

Shock: Initial assessment by determining the number of hours (≥2) that patients spent in each of the following categories. The worst category attained during the first 24 hours was noted for each patient

Systolic blood pressure (mm Hg)	Heart rate			
	<60	60–100	101–149	≥ 150
<90	Possibly yes	Possibly yes	Probably yes	Probably yes
90–200	Probably not	Probably not	Possibly yes	Possibly yes
>200	Not shock	Not shock	Not shock	Not shock

Final shock categories were determined by:

1. Raising the initial shock category from "possible yes" to "probably yes" if the patient was on continuous vasoactive drugs for 1 hour or more or if the cardiac index was less than 2.5 or more than 4.5 L/min/m² at any time during the first 24 hours.
2. Lowering the initial shock category one level ("possibly yes" became "probably not") if the cardiac index was 2.5–4.5 L/min/m² (exception: if the patient was on vasoactive drugs, the initial shock category was raised one level, as in 1).

2. Multiply the value in column A for your patient by column B; then add up the total points.

Variable	Column A	Column B	Subtotals
Constant	1	−3.0	−3.0
Level of consciousness			
Coma or deep stupor	1	2.63	
Neither coma nor deep stupor	0		
Type of admission			
Emergency	1	1.63	
Elective	0		
Cancer			
Yes	1	1.49	
No	0		
Infection			
Yes	1	0.677	
No	0		
No. of organ system failures	#	0.595	
Age (years)	Years	0.038	
Systolic blood pressure (SBP)	SBP	−0.048	
Systolic blood pressure squared	SBP^2	0.000131	
		Total:	

3. Estimate the probability of dying in the hospital (“Factor” is the total from step 2 above).

$$\text{Probability of dying in the hospital } (0\text{–}1) = e^{\text{Factor}}/(1 + e^{\text{Factor}})$$

4. You can also estimate the probability of dying in the hospital from the table below.

Total from Step 2	Probability of dying in-hospital
−12 to −6	0%
−5	1%
−4	2%
−3	5%
−2	12%
−1	27%
0	50%
1	73%
2	88%
3	95%
4	98%
5	99%
≥6	100%

Probability of Death from Burn Injuries

Clinical question

What is the probability of in-hospital death for patients with burn injuries?

Population and setting

Consecutive patients admitted to the Shriners Burn Institute and Massachusetts General Hospital between 1990 and 1994 were used to develop the rule and those admitted in 1995 and 1996 to test it. Of the 1665 patients in the training group, 910 (55%) were children, 69% were male, and the mean age was 21 years (range 1 month to 99 years). A group of 244 patients (15%) had an inhalation injury, and 8% required escharotomy. The mean length of hospital stay was 21 days.

Study size

The training group had 1665 patients and the validation group 530 patients.

Pretest probability

Four percent of patients died.

Type of validation

Grade II: The validation group was a separate sample from the same population, with data for the validation group gathered prospectively.

Comments

This is a well validated rule. Results were similar for application of the rule to the training and validation groups, so both are reported below.

Reference

Ryan CM, Schoenfeld DA, Thorpe WP, et al. Objective estimates of the pretest probability of death from burn injuries. N Engl J Med 1998;338:362–366.

CLINICAL PREDICTION RULE

1. Count the number of risk factors your patients has.

Risk factor	Points
Age >60 years	1
Burn covering more than 40% of the body surface area (BSA)	1
Inhalation injury	1
Total:	

2. The risk of death in the training and validation groups is shown below.

		Mortality rate	
No. of risk factors	No. of patients	Training group	Validation group
0	1314	0.2%	0.7%
1	218	5.0%	14.0%
2	111	30.0%	39.0%
3	22	95.0%	90.0%

3. The length of stay for survivors can be estimated below (data from training group).

BSA burned	Length of stay (days)	No. of patients
<20%	6–17	1295
20–39%	17–45	187
40–89%	38–94	104
≥90%	129–237	12

Mortality Based on Number of Organ System Failures

Clinical question

What is the patient's prognosis based on the number of organ system failures?

Population and setting

Consecutive patients admitted to a French intensive care unit (ICU) between 1987 and 1990 were included. The mean age was 55 years; 65% were male. The mean APACHE II score was 19, and the mean SAPS score was 13.

Study size

Altogether, 1070 patients were studied.

Pretest probability

Among the patients, 26.7% died.

Type of validation

Grade IV: The training group was used as the validation group.

Comments

This rule has not been prospectively validated. However, the idea of the number of organ systems being related to the prognosis is a common one in the ICU and has good face validity. This provides preliminary evidence that it has true validity. However, more studies are needed.

Reference

Fagon JY, Chastre J, Novara A, Medioni P, Gibert C. Characterization of intensive care unit patients using a model based on the presence or absence of organ dysfunctions and/or infection: the ODIN model. Intensive Care Med 1993;19:137–144.

CLINICAL PREDICTION RULE

1. Count the number of organ system failures for your patient, using the following definitions.

Organ system	Definition	Points
Pulmonary	One or more of the following	1
	$PaO_2 < 60$ mm Hg on $FIO_2 = 0.21$	
	Need for ventilatory support	
Cardiovascular	One or more of the following, in the absence of hypovolemia	1
	Systolic arterial pressure < 90 mm Hg with signs of peripheral hypoperfusion	
	Continuous infusion of vasopressor or inotropic agents required to maintain systolic pressure > 90 mm Hg	
Renal	One or more of the following	1
	Serum creatinine > 300 μmol/L	
	Urine output <500 ml/24 hr or < 180 ml/8 hr	
	Need for hemodialysis or peritoneal dialysis	
Neurologic	One or more of the following	1
	Glasgow Coma Scale ≤ 6 (in the absence of sedation at any one point in the day)	
	Sudden onset of confusion or psychosis	
Hepatic	One or more of the following	1
	Serum bilirubin > 100 μmol/L	
	Alkaline phosphatase more than three times normal	
Hematologic	One or more of the following	1
	Hematocrit ≤ 20%	
	White blood cell count < $2000/mm^3$	
	Platelet count < $40,000/mm^3$	
Infection	One or more of the following associated with clinical evidence of infection	1
	Two or more positive blood cultures	
	Presence of gross pus in a closed space	
	Source of the infection determined during hospitalization or at autopsy in case of death within 24 hours	
	Total (0–7):	

2. The probability of in-hospital death is shown below.

No. of organ dysfunctions	Survivors (no.)	Nonsurvivors (no.)	Survivors	Likelihood ratio for survival
0	148	4	97%	13.5
1	214	23	90%	3.4
2	239	48	83%	1.8
3	128	61	68%	0.8
4	39	72	35%	0.2
5	14	44	24%	0.1
6	2	29	6%	0.03
7	0	5	0%	0

4

Dermatology

■ RISK OF PRESSURE SORES (BRADEN SCALE)

Risk of Pressure Sores in Nursing Home Patients

Clinical question

Which patients in a nursing home are at risk for the development of pressure sores?

Population and setting

A random sample of patients admitted to a nursing home within 72 hours who did not have pressure sores were included. Patients were evaluated every 2–3 days for 4 weeks.

Study size

Altogether, 102 patients were studied.

Pretest probability

Of these patients, 27.5% developed a pressure sore during the first 4 weeks of the study.

Type of validation

Grade I: The validation group was from a distinct population. The rule was developed in one group of patients and validated in another.

Comments

Not surprisingly, the Braden score becomes more accurate as you get closer to the appearance of the pressure sore. Note also that the cutpoints in each study were chosen post hoc by the investigators, after examination of the data. A different cutpoint may be more appropriate in your setting. Although the scale is somewhat subjective, it has good interrater reliability (88% agreement) when used by skilled nurse clinicians.

References

Bergstrom N, Braden B, Boynton P, Bruch S. Using a research-based assessment scale in clinical practice. Nurs Clin North Am 1995;30:539–551.

Bergstrom N, Braden B, Kemp M, Champagne M, Ruby E. Multi-site study of incidence of pressure ulcers and the relationship between risk level, demographic characteristics, diagnoses, and prescription of preventive interventions. J Am Geriatr Soc 1996;44:22–30.

Braden BJ, Bergstrom N. Predictive validity of the Braden Scale for pressure sore risk in a nursing home population. Res Nurs Health 1994;17:459–470.

Jiricka MK, Ryan P, Carvalho MA, Bukvich J. Pressure ulcer risk factors in an ICU population. Am J Crit Care 1995;4:361–367.

CLINICAL PREDICTION RULE

1. Calculate your patient's Braden Score (range 6–23).

Risk factor	Description	Points
Sensory perception (able to respond meaningfully to pressure-related discomfort)		
No impairment	Responds to verbal commands. Has no sensory deficit that would limit ability to feel or voice pain or discomfort.	4
Slightly limited	Responds to verbal commands but cannot always communicate discomfort or need to be turned. Also may have some sensory impairment that limits ability to feel pain or discomfort in one or two extremities.	3
Very limited	Responds only to painful stimuli and cannot communicate discomfort except by moaning or restlessness. Also may have sensory impairment that limits the ability to feel pain or discomfort over half of the body.	2
Completely limited	Unresponsive to painful stimuli. Also may have limited ability to feel pain over most of body surface.	1
Moisture (degree to which skin is exposed to moisture)		
Rarely moist	Skin is usually dry, and linen requires changing only at routine intervals.	4
Occasionally moist	Skin is occasionally moist, requiring an extra linen change about once a day.	3
Very moist	Skin is often but not always moist.	2
Constantly moist	Skin is kept moist almost constantly.	1
Activity (degree of physical activity)		
Walks frequently	Walks outside of room at least twice a day and inside room.	4
Walks occasionally	Walks occasionally during day but for very short distances, with or without assistance.	3
Chair-bound	Ability to walk severely limited or nonexistent.	2
Bed-bound	Confined to bed.	1
Mobility (ability to change and control body position)		
No limitations	Makes major and frequent changes in position without assistance.	4
Slightly limited	Makes frequent though slight changes in body or extremity position independently.	3
Very limited	Makes occasional slight changes in body or extremity but unable to make significant changes independently.	2
Completely immobile	Does not make even slight changes in body or extremity position without assistance.	1

Risk factor	Description	Points
Nutrition (usual food intake pattern)		
Excellent	Eats most of every meal and never refuses a meal.	4
Adequate	Eats over half of most meals and may occasionally refuse a meal.	3
Probably inadequate	Rarely eats a complete meal and has decreased protein intake.	2
Very poor	Never eats a complete meal and rarely eats more than one-third of food offered. Also if NPO or on clear fluid or intravenous infusions for more than 5 days.	1
Shear and friction		
No problem apparent	Moves in bed and in chair independently and has sufficient muscle strength to lift up completely during move.	3
Potential problem	Moves feebly or requires minimum assistance.	2
Problem present	Requires moderate to maximum assistance in moving; complete lifting without sliding against sheets is impossible.	1
	Total:	

2. The risk of a pressure ulcer can be determined with this table.

Patient population and timing of Braden Score	Cutoff[a]	Sensitivity/specificity	LR^+	LR^-
Nursing home				
On admission	≤18	75%/59%	1.8	0.4
3 Days after admission	≤18	79%/68%	2.5	0.3
3 Days before diagnosis of pressure ulcer	≤18	79%/74%	3.0	0.3
Acute hospital bed	≤16	100%/90%	10	0.01

[a]Less than or equal to this number is defined as abnormal and at risk for pressure ulcer.
LR^+ = positive likelihood ratio; LR^- = negative likelihood ratio.

Risk of Pressure Sores (Norton Scale)

Clinical question

What is the risk of pressure sores in a hospitalized elderly population?

Population and setting

The rule was developed and tested in the geriatric unit of an English hospital. Demographic data are not available.

Study size

The rule was evaluated in 250 patients.

Pretest probability

Of these patients, 24% developed a pressure sore.

Type of validation

Not clear from the study.

Comments

It is not clear how the rule was validated. It appears to have been developed and then tested on the 250 patients for whom data are here reported. A prospective study of 218 patients for whom data are not reported was said to give similar results according to the authors. The major limitations of the rule are the questionable validation and the lack of clear definitions of the physical condition and mental condition variables.

Reference

Norton D. Calculating the risk: reflections on the Norton Scale. Decubitus 1989;2:24–30.

CLINICAL PREDICTION RULE

1. Calculate the patient's risk score. The risk score should be recalculated as the patient progresses through the hospital stay.

Variable	Points
Physical condition	
Good	4
Fair	3
Poor	2
Very bad	1
Mental condition	
Alert	4
Apathetic	3
Confused	2
Stupor	1
Activity	
Ambulant	4
Walk/help	3
Chairbound	2
Bed	1
Mobility	
Full	4
Slightly limited	3
Very limited	2
Immobile	1
Incontinent	
Not	4
Occasional	3
Usually/urine	2
Doubly (urine and stool)	1
Total:	

2. The risk of a pressure sore is shown below.

Initial risk score	With pressure sore
<12	48%
12–14	32%
15–17	21%
18–20	5%

5

Endocrinology

METABOLIC PROBLEMS

Differential Diagnosis of Hypercalcemia

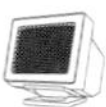

Clinical question

What is the differential diagnosis of hypercalcemia, specifically malignancy versus primary hypoparathyroidism?

Population studied

All patients with an albumin-adjusted calcium value ≥2.7 mmol/L at a Scottish hospital were included.

Study size

Altogether, 148 patients were studied.

Pretest probability

Hypercalcemia was caused by primary hypoparathyroidism in 76 patients, malignancy in 53, and other causes in 19.

Type of validation

Grade IV: The training group was used as the validation group.

Comments

This rule should be used with caution, as it has not been prospectively validated. Also, we are given no demographic information about the patients other than their final diagnoses.

Reference

Gibb JA, Ogston SA, Paterson CR, Evans JU. Discriminant functions in differential diagnosis of hypercalcemic patients. Clin Chem 1990;36:358–361.

CLINICAL PREDICTION RULE

Definitions

Albumin = grams per liter
Phosphate = millimoles per liter
GGT = γ-glutamyl transferase (units per liter)
Chloride = millimoles per liter
Ca_{exc} = calcium excretion (millimoles/liter)

1. Calculate your patient's score from the following formula.

$$\text{Score} = (0.1265 \times \text{albumin}) - (1.498 \times \text{phosphate}) + (0.1194 \times \text{chloride}) - [1.325 \times \log_{10} (Ca_{exc})] - [0.9321 \times \log_{10} (\text{GGT})] - 15.11$$

2. Find your patient's probability of primary hypoparathyroidism and malignancy.

Score	% With this score who have primary hypoparathyroidism	% With this score who have malignancy	% With primary hypoparathyroidism who have this score	% With malignancy who have this score
>0	86.0	14.0	97.4	22.6
≤0	5.7	95.3	2.6	77.4

DIABETES MELLITUS

Screening for Diabetes Mellitus

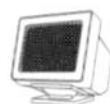

Clinical question

What is the likelihood of diabetes mellitus among patients presenting for screening?

Population and setting

A random sample of patients aged 20–79 years, selected from the general population to be representative of the U.S. population by age, race, and gender, were included. All reported having no history of diabetes. Diabetes was diagnosed based on a glucose tolerance test.

Study size

Altogether, 3384 patients were studied.

Pretest probability

Of these patients, 4.8% had diabetes mellitus by World Health Organization (WHO) criteria.

Type of validation

Grade IV: The training group was used as the validation group.

Comments

This study has the strength of using a large, representative, population-based sample. However, it has not yet been validated on a new set of patients and should be used only with caution.

Reference

Herman VH, Engelgau MM, Smith PJ, et al. A new and simple questionnaire to identify people at increased risk for undiagnosed diabetes. Diabetes Care 1995;18:382–387.

CLINICAL PREDICTION RULE

Definitions

Obesity = weight for height ≥ 120% ideal body weight for medium frame

Sedentary = little or no exercise during recreation and quite inactive during a usual day

The classification tree indicates groups at high risk (>5%) of undiagnosed diabetes mellitus in boldface. The tree has a sensitivity of 83%, specificity of 65%, and positive predictive value of 11%; the area under the receiver-operating characteristic (ROC) curve is 0.78.

Screening For Diabetes

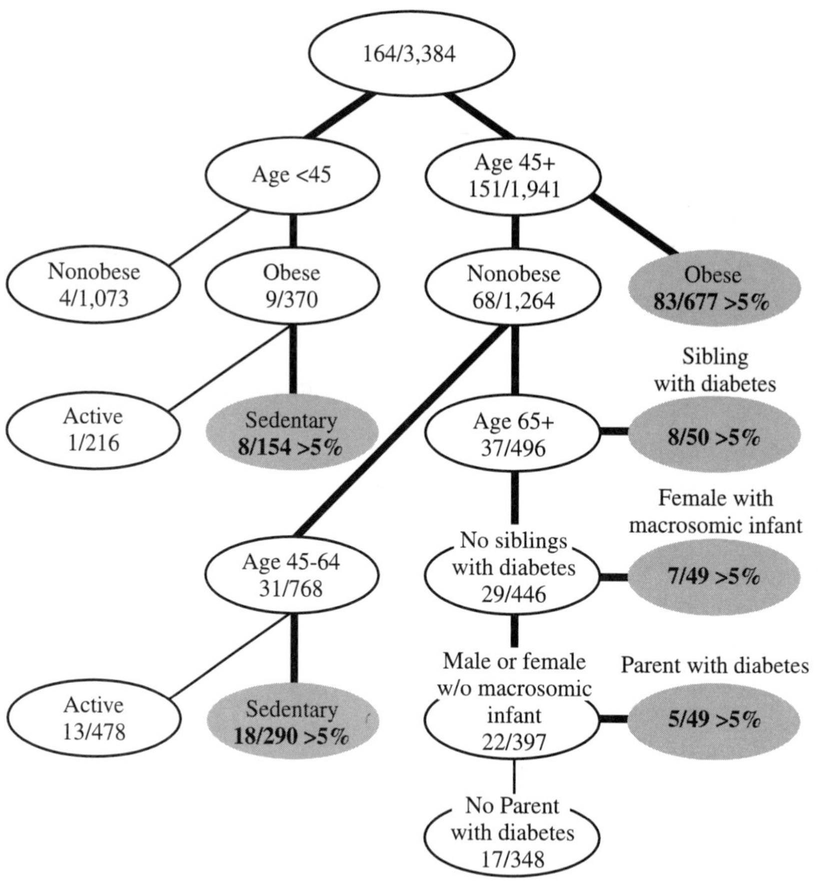

Insulin-Dependent or Non-Insulin-Dependent Diabetes Mellitus?

Clinical question

Does a patient presenting with new onset diabetes mellitus have insulin-dependent or non-insulin-dependent disease?

Population and setting

The authors studied 281 patients enrolled in the Rochester Diabetic Neuropathy study. The C-peptide response 6 minutes after intravenous glucagon injection was the reference standard for the diagnosis of insulin-dependent diabetes mellitus (IDDM). Patients were roughly 50% male; the age of onset for IDDM was 19.2 years and for NIDDM 55.1 years.

Study size

The validation group had 346 patients.

Pretest probability

Altogether, 84 patients had IDDM and 262 had NIDDM.

Type of validation

Grade I: The validation group was from a distinct population. The rule was developed in one group of patients and validated in another.

Comments

This rule shows that it is possible to use the history and physical examination alone to make a reasonably accurate diagnosis of the type of diabetes mellitus. This information can be useful when initially counseling patients.

Reference

Service EJ, Rizza RA, Zimmerman BR, et al. The classification of diabetes by clinical and C-peptide criteria. Diabetes Care 1997;20:198–201.

CLINICAL PREDICTION RULE

Use this algorithm to determine whether your patient with newly diagnosed diabetes has non-insulin-dependent diabetes mellitus (NIDDM) or insulin-dependent diabetes mellitus (IDDM).

+ = positive
PR = physician review

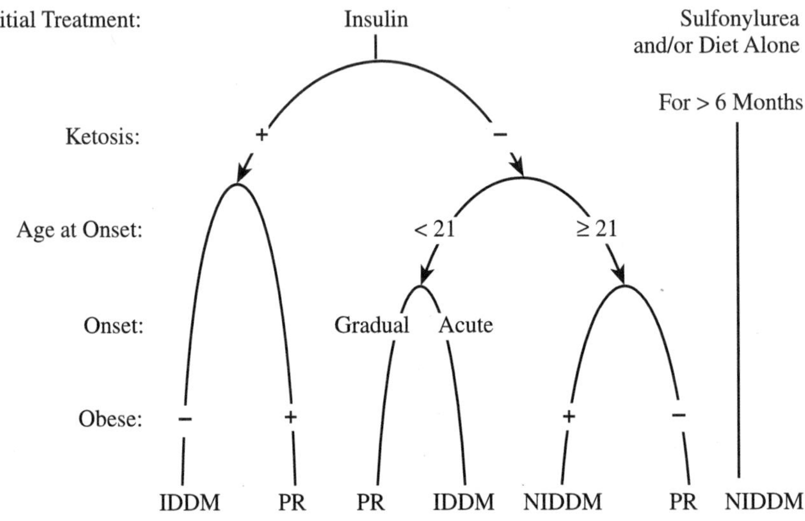

6

ENT/Ophthalmology

CATARACT SURGERY

Likelihood of Benefit from Cataract Surgery

Clinical question

Which patients over age 65 undergoing cataract surgery will benefit from the procedure?

Population and setting

Consecutive patients over age 65 scheduled for their first or second cataract surgery at the Massachusetts Eye and Ear Institute were included. Patients from 33 general ophthalmology practices in the Boston area were also included. Patients were excluded if they could not communicate with the research staff, refused to participate, or their surgery was cancelled (264 of 690 patients were excluded for these reasons). The mean age was 76.6 years, and 69% were female.

Study size

There were 281 patients in the training group and 145 in the validation group.

Pretest probability

Among these patients, 39% had substantial improvement, 20% some improvement, and 41% minimal or no improvement.

Type of validation

Grade III: The validation group was a separate sample from the same population, although data for both training and validation groups were gathered at the same time.

Comments

Note that the Activities of Daily Vision Scale (ADVS) score is used as both a predictor variable and for the outcome. This inflates the accuracy of the model. Otherwise it was a fairly well designed rule.

Reference

Mangione CM, Orav EJ, Lawrence MG, Phillips RS, Seddon JM, Goldman L. Prediction of visual function after cataract surgery: a prospectively validated model. Arch Ophthalmol 1995;113:1305–1311.

CLINICAL PREDICTION RULE

1. Add points for your patient (note that the presence of posterior subcapsular changes results in *subtracting* a point).

Variable	Points
Age	
65–74	1
75–84	2
85–94	3
>94	4
Preoperative ADVS score	+(0.1 × ADVS)
Posterior subcapsular changes	−1 if present
Macular degeneration	+1 if present
Diabetes mellitus	+2 if present
Total:	

ADVS = Activities of Daily Vision Scale.

2. Find the patient outcome based on the total score.

Score	Substantial Improvement	Some improvement	No/minimal Improvement
≤6	85%	3%	12%
7–10	34%	34%	32%
>10	3%	12%	85%

HEARING IMPAIRMENT

Hearing Handicap Inventory for the Elderly: Screening Version

Clinical question

Is this elderly patient hearing impaired?

Population and setting

Consecutive patients over age 65 presenting to an internist's office. All patients who agreed to both screening and audiometry were included. The mean age was 74 years; 77% were white; and 63% were female.

Study size

Altogether, 178 patients were used to validate the rule.

Pretest probability

Of these patients, 30% were hearing-impaired (40 db loss at the 1000- or 2000-Hz frequency in both ears or a 40 db loss at the 1000- and 2000-Hz frequencies in one ear).

Type of validation

Grade I: The validation group was from a distinct population. The rule was developed in one group of patients and validated in another.

Comments

This rule is practical and useful; and it was well validated in a primary care population. Note that the simple whispered voice test at 2 feet has excellent sensitivity (100%) and adequate specificity (84%) as a more rapid screen.

References

Lichtenstein MJ, Bess FH, Logan SA. Validation of screening tools for identifying hearing-impaired elderly in primary care. JAMA 1988;259:2875–2878.
MacPhee GF, Crowther JA, McAlpine CH. Age Ageing 1988;17:347–351.

CLINICAL PREDICTION RULE

1. Add up the number of points for your patient.

Question (possible responses are "no," "sometimes," or "yes")	No	Sometimes	Yes
Does a hearing problem cause you to feel embarrassed when you meet new people?	0	2	4
Does a hearing problem cause you to feel frustrated when talking to members of your family?	0	2	4
Do you have difficulty hearing when someone speaks in a whisper?	0	2	4
Do you feel handicapped by a hearing problem?	0	2	4
Does a hearing problem cause you difficulty when visiting friends, relatives, or neighbors?	0	2	4
Does a hearing problem cause you to attend religious services less often than you would like?	0	2	4
Does a hearing problem cause you to have arguments with family members?	0	2	4
Does a hearing problem cause you difficulty when listening to television or radio?	0	2	4
Do you feel that any difficulty with your hearing limits hampers your personal or social life?	0	2	4
Does a hearing problem cause you difficulty when in a restaurant with relatives or friends?	0	2	4
Total:			

"No" = 0; "sometimes" = 2; and "yes" = 4.

2. Interpret their score below (post-test probabilities assume a baseline risk of 30% for hearing impairment):

Score	Likelihood ratio	Probability of hearing impairment
0–8	0.2	13%
9–24	2.3	50%
25–40	12.0	84%

7

Gastroenterology

PEPTIC ULCER DISEASE AND DYSPEPSIA

Ulcer in Patients with Dyspepsia

Clinical question

What is the likelihood of peptic ulcer among outpatients with dyspepsia?

Population and setting

Adult dyspeptic patients referred from English general practices to a gastroenterology clinic for endoscopy were included.

Study size

The training group included 560 patients and the validation group 550.

Pretest probability

The prevalence of ulcer was 38% in the training group and 44% in the validation group. This is higher than in the average primary care setting because these patients were selected by their general practitioner for endoscopy.

Type of validation

Grade III: The validation group was a separate sample from the same population, although data for both training and validation groups were gathered at the same time.

Comments

There is some potential for misinterpretation of several of the predictor variables, such as "episodic pain," "lost appetite," and "flatulence." (Who is not flatulent at some time?) Also, demographic information was not reported. The methods were otherwise solid; and although somewhat complex, this is probably the best score for predicting ulcer in dyspeptic patients.

Reference

Spiegelhalter DJ, Crean GP, Holden R, Knill-Jones RP. Taking a calculated risk: predictive scoring systems in dyspepsia. J Scand Gastroenterol 1987;128(suppl):152–160.

CLINICAL PREDICTION RULE

1. Add up the number of points for your patient.

Variable	Points
Male gender	
Yes	30
No	−33
Main symptom pain	
Yes	13
No	−27
Length of history < 2 years	
Yes	38
No	−40
Episodic pain	
Yes	13
No	−25
Pain in epigastrium	
Yes	26
No	−29
Food reduces pain	
Yes	72
No	−22
Night waking + food relief	
Yes	51
No	−23
Vomiting	
Yes	5
No	−2
Waterbrash (bitter taste in back of mouth/throat)	
Yes	38
No	−18
Flatulence	
Yes	4
No	−5
Lost appetite	
Yes	18
No	−14
Family history of ulcer	
Yes	24
No	−15
Smoker	
Yes	31
No	−51
Heartburn	
Yes	5
No	−8
Total:	

2. The probability of ulcer is calculated using the following formula.

$$\text{Probability of ulcer} = e^{(\text{score}/100)}/[1 + e^{(\text{score}/100)}]$$

Using a cutoff of 0, the score has 71% sensitivity and 83% specificity.

3. The probability of ulcer for various scores can also be found below. Remember that this assumes an underlying rate of ulcer around 40%, and the typical primary care rate is closer to 25%.

Score	Probability of ulcer
−300	5%
−250	8%
−200	12%
−150	18%
−125	22%
−100	27%
−75	32%
−50	38%
−25	44%
0	50%
25	56%
50	62%
75	68%
100	73%
125	78%
150	82%
200	88%
250	92%
300	95%

GASTROINTESTINAL HEMORRHAGE

Likelihood of Gastrointestinal Bleeding in the Intensive Care Unit

Clinical question

What is the likelihood of gastrointestinal (GI) bleeding in critically ill patients?

Population and setting

Consecutive patients over age 16 admitted to the intensive care unit (ICU) at one of four university hospitals were included. Patients were excluded if there was evidence of upper GI bleeding within 48 hours before or 24 hours after admission to the ICU, brain death, facial trauma, hopeless prognosis, or if they died or were discharged within 24 hours of admission. The mean age was 60 years, and 66% were male. Diagnoses included cardiovascular surgery (48.5%), respiratory disease (12.1%), gastrointestinal disease (9.8%), and cardiovascular disease (6.3%).

Study size

A total of 2252 patients were studied.

Pretest probability

Of these patients, 4.4% had overt bleeding episodes (87 of 100 were receiving prophylaxis against stress ulcers).

Type of validation

Grade IV: The training group was used as the validation group.

Comments

This simple rule identifies a large group of ICU patients who are at low risk of bleeding, and from whom prophylaxis against stress ulcers can safely be withheld. The main limitation is the lack of prospective validation, so it should be used with some caution.

Reference

Cook DJ, Fuller HD, Guyatt GH, et al. Risk factors for gastrointestinal bleeding in critically ill patients. N Engl J Med 1994;330:377–381.

CLINICAL PREDICTION RULE

Patients who did not undergo mechanical ventilation for more than 48 hours *and* who had no coagulopathy (62% of patients) had a low risk of bleeding (0.1%).

Mortality Associated with Upper Gastrointestinal Bleeding

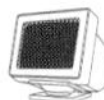

Clinical question

What is the mortality following acute upper gastrointestinal (GI) bleeding?

Population and setting

The authors included all identified patients at British hospitals in four health regions with acute GI bleeding over a 4-month period in 1993 (training group) and a 4-month period in 1994 (validation group). In the training group, 1294 of 4185 were under 60 years old, 1754 were 60–79 years old, and 1094 were 80 years or older; 57% were male. Final diagnoses included peptic ulcer in 1450, malignancy in 155, Mallory-Weiss tear in 214, erosive disease in 447, esophagitis in 429, varices in 180, and no or other diagnosis in 1267.

Study size

There were 4185 patients in the training group and 1625 in the validation group.

Pretest probability

Altogether, 18.7% experienced rebleeding, and 14.5% died.

Type of validation

Grade I: The validation group was from a distinct population. The rule was developed in one group of patients and validated in another.

Comments

This is a well designed, useful clinical rule. The only quibbles are the question of generalizability to American patients and the lack of clear definitions for comorbidities, such as renal disease, ischemic heart disease, and congestive heart failure.

Reference

Rockall TA, Logan RF, Develin HB, et al. Risk assessment after acute upper gastrointestinal haemorrhage. Gut 1996;38:316–321.

CLINICAL PREDICTION RULE

1. The history-only score uses adds the points from the first 3 rows of the table (age, shock, comorbidity) and has a maximum of 7. The full score requiring endoscopy uses all five rows and has a maximum of 11.

	Score			
Variable	0	1	2	3
History only variables				
Age	< 60 Years	60–79 Years	≥ 80 Years	—
Shock	No shock: SBP ≥ 100 mm Hg and pulse < 100 bpm	Tachycardia: SBP ≥ 100 mm Hg and pulse ≥ 100 bpm	Hypotension: SBP < 100 mm Hg	—
Co-morbidity	No Major co-morbidity	—	CHF, ischemic heart disease, any other major co-morbidity	Renal failure, liver failure, or disseminated cancer
Variables requiring endoscopy				
Diagnosis	Mallory-Weiss tear, no lesion identified, no SRH	All others	Malignancy of upper GI tract	—
SRH	None or dark spot only	—	Blood in upper GI tract, adherent clot, visible or spurting vessel	—

SBP = systolic blood pressure; CHF = congestive heart failure; SRH = stigmata of recent hemorrhage; GI = gastrointestinal.

2. Interpreting the history-only score (no endoscopy, maximum = 7).

Parameter	0	1	2	3	4	5	6	7
No. of patients in group	246	201	249	311	364	134	68	8
Deaths	0%	3.0%	6.1%	12.1%	21.0%	35.1%	61.8%	75.0%

3. Interpreting the full score (with endoscopy, maximum = 11).

Parameter	0	1	2	3	4	5	6	7	≥ 8
No. of patients in group	48	131	142	162	176	199	137	106	89
Rebleeding	4.2%	4.6%	7.7%	11.7%	15.3%	24.6%	27.0%	36.8%	37.1%
Deaths	0%	0%	0%	1.8%	7.9%	10.6%	11.7%	22.6%	40.4%

Adverse Events with Upper Gastrointestinal Hemorrhage

Clinical question

What is the risk of adverse events in patients with upper gastrointestinal (UGI) hemorrhage?

Population and setting

In the retrospective chart review evaluation, adult patients hospitalized between January 1992 and June 30, 1993, admitted to Cedars Sinai Medical Center for an admitting or primary diagnosis of gastrointestinal hemorrhage based on ICD-9 codes were included. Patients without complete medical records were excluded. The prospective evaluation included adult patients admitted to the same hospital between May 1994 and July 1995 for hematemesis, nasogastric tube aspirate containing gross or occult blood, or a history of hematemesis or melena and diagnostic endoscopy.

Study size

Retrospective chart review: 500 patients were studied. Prospective evaluation: 299 patients were identified, of whom 209 met low risk criteria.

Pretest probability

Retrospective evaluation: in-hospital mortality was 6.8%; 6.4% required emergency surgery; and 30.8% experienced recurrent bleeding after hospitalization. A total of 19.0% experienced a life-threatening event (death, emergency GI surgery, or major rebleeding).

Type of validation

Grade I: The rule was developed from a review of the literature and was validated in an independent population.

Comments

The retrospective validation used a chart review, and the prospective validation gathered new data but only followed low risk patients. This clinical rule forms the basis for a clinical practice guideline used at Cedars Sinai Hospital in Los Angeles. It is important to review both articles in detail before applying this clinical guideline in your institution.

References

Hay JA, Lyubashevsky E, Elashoff J, et al. Upper gastrointestinal hemorrhage clinical guidelines: determining the optimum hospital length of stay. Am J Med 1996; 100:313–322.

Hay JA, Maldonado L, Weingarten SR, Ellrodt AG. Prospective evaluation of a clinical guideline recommending hospital length of stay in upper gastrointestinal tract hemorrhage. JAMA 1997;278:2151–2156.

CLINICAL PREDICTION RULE

1. Calculate the risk score.

EGD Risk factor	Points
Findings	
PUD without SRH, nonbleeding M-W tear, erosive disease, or normal EGD[a]	0
PUD with spot or clot, erosive disease with SRH, or angiodysplasia	1
PUD with visible vessel (nonbleeding) or SRH[b]	2
Persistent UGI hemorrhage, varices, or carcinoma	4
Time	
48 hours	0
<48 hours	1
In hospital	2
Hemodynamics	
Stable	0
Intermediate	1
Unstable	2
No. of co-morbidities[a]	
≤1	0
2	1
3	2
≥4	3
Total:	

PUD = peptic ulcer disease; M-W = Mallory-Weiss; NB = nonbleeding; VVNB = visible vessel, nonbleeding; SRH = stigmata of recent hemorrhage; EGD = esophagogastroduodenoscopy

[a]Clinician should consider aortoenteric fistula if the patient presents with hemodynamic instability and normal EGD findings.

[b]Presence of stigmata of recent hemorrhage not specified by the endoscopist.

[c]Possible co-morbidities:

- Cardiac disease; dysrhythmia, acute myocardial infarction, ischemic chest pain (symptomatic and requiring treatment), congestive heart failure
- Hepatic disease: acute alcoholic hepatitis, cirrhosis
- Pulmonary disease: acute respiratory failure, pneumonia, obstructive lung disease
- Renal disease: serum creatinine > 4 mg/dl, dialysis therapy
- Neurologic disease: delirium, dementia, stroke within 6 months
- Malignancy: known solid tumor
- Sepsis
- Major surgery within 30 days
- Age > 60 years
- Unstable co-morbidity: meets criteria for continued in-hospital treatment

2. Interpret the score.

		Prognosis (risk of life-threatening complications)	
Score	Risk category	Retrospective chart review	Prospective validation
0–2	Low	0% (0–2.2%)	0% (0–0.9%)
3–4	Intermediate	9.1% (5.2–13.0%)	NA
>4	High	45.5% (37.9–53.1%)	NA

Numbers in parentheses are the 95% confidence interval.

Mortality Due to Variceal Bleeding

Clinical question

What is the likelihood of death during the first 6 weeks after the initial presentation of variceal bleeding in a cirrhotic patient?

Population and setting

Patients with an initial episode of variceal bleeding between June 1983 and December 1988 were included. Those with incomplete records, prehepatic portal hypertension, hepatocellular carcinoma, or other neoplasm were excluded (19 total). All had hepatic cirrhosis, of whom 63% had alcoholic cirrhosis.

Study size

Altogether, 102 patients were studied.

Pretest probability

Of these patients, 28% died within the first 6 weeks and 40% at 1 year.

Type of validation

Grade IV: The training group was used as the validation group.

Comments

This study provides some guidance regarding the prognosis of patients presenting with an initial episode of esophageal variceal bleeding. It should be prospectively validated in your setting before application to patient care.

Reference

Le Moine O, Bourgeois N, Delhaye M, et al. Factors related to early mortality in cirrhotic patients bleeding from varices and treated by urgent sclerotherapy. Gut 1992;33:1381–1385.

CLINICAL PREDICTION RULE

Definitions

ENC = encephalopathy (1 if absent, 2 if moderate, 3 if coma)

PT = prothrombin time (absolute value in seconds)

BU = number of blood units transfused within 72 hours after identification of variceal bleeding

1. Calculate the score.

$$\text{Score} = (2.75 \times \text{ENC}) + (0.1 \times \text{PT}) - (0.31 \times \text{BU}) + 2.64$$

2. Estimate the probability of dying at 6 weeks.

$$\text{Probability of dying at 6 weeks} = e^{\text{Score}}/(e^{\text{Score}} + 1)$$

3. You can also use the table below, once you have calculated the score.

Score	Probability of dying at 6 weeks
≤−6	0%
−5	1%
−4	2%
−3	5%
−2	12%
−1	27%
0	50%
1	73%
2	88%
3	95%
4	98%
5	99%
≥6	100%

In the original study, 71 of 73 patients with a score <0.7 survived at least 6 weeks, and 16 of 18 patients with a score >0.7 died by 6 weeks.

Continued Upper Gastrointestinal Bleeding after Endoscopic Injection

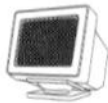

Clinical question

Which patients with bleeding peptic ulcer will have persistent bleeding after endoscopic injection?

Population and setting

All patients admitted to a Spanish teaching hospital because of upper gastrointestinal (GI) bleeding with peptic ulcer who had active arterial bleeding (spurting or oozing) at endoscopy were included. The mean age was 65 years; 66% were male.

Study size

The training group had 233 patients and the validation group 88.

Pretest probability

Of patients in the validation group, 23% had a therapeutic failure of endoscopic injection.

Type of validation

Grade II: The validation group was a separate sample from the same population, with data for the validation group gathered prospectively.

Comments

Although this study has the strength of prospective validation, the validation group is relatively small. There are the additional issues of generalizability from Spain to other populations and ambiguity in some of the predictor variables such as "associated diseases."

Reference

Villanueva C, Balanzo J, Espinos JC, et al. Prediction of therapeutic failure in patients with bleeding peptic ulcer treated with endoscopic injection. Dig Dis Sci 1993;38: 2062–2070.

CLINICAL PREDICTION RULE

1. Review the following definitions.

Patients are considered to have "associated disease" if they have any of the following conditions: chronic illnesses such as a past medical history of cardiovascular, respiratory, hepatic, renal, oncologic, metabolic, or rheumatologic disease deemed clinically significant, or any disorders identified as an active problem requiring close attention at the time of admission, such as pneumonia or acute renal failure.

SWB = superior wall of the duodenal bulb.

PWB = posterior wall of the duodenal bulb.

2. The likelihood of recurrent bleeding is shown below, based on the patient's ulcer size, site, and if there is an "associated disease" as defined above.

	Percent, by ulcer size (5–30 mm)							
	No associated disease				Associated disease			
Ulcer site	5 mm	10 mm	20 mm	30 mm	5 mm	10 mm	20 mm	30 mm
SWB	37%	43%	56%	68%	60%	66%	77%	85%
PWB	28%	34%	46%	59%	51%	57%	69%	79%
Other	4%	5%	8%	13%	9%	12%	19%	29%

GALLBLADDER AND PANCREATIC DISEASE

Likelihood of Common Bile Duct Lithiasis

Clinical question

Which patients undergoing choecystectomy for symptomatic cholelithiasis are at risk for common bile duct lithiasis (CBDL)?

Population and setting

All patients undergoing cholecystectomy for symptomatic cholelithiasis at one of four surgical units in France were included. The mean age was 60.4 years (range 18–91 years); 75% were women. Data were collected prospectively. Patients with cirrhosis, incidental cholecystectomy, or biliary tumor and patients being operated for retained stones after cholecystectomy were excluded.

Study size

The training group consisted of 503 patients and the validation group 279.

Pretest probability

The probability of a CBDL was 15% in the validation group.

Type of validation

Grade II: The validation group was a separate sample from the same population, with data for the validation group gathered prospectively.

Comments

Most patients in this study underwent laparoscopic cholecystectomy. The high rate of CBDL in the group with a "positive" score (39%) suggests that routine exploration, further study, or both may be indicated in these patients.

Reference

Houdart R, Perniceni T, Dame B, et al. Predicting common bile duct lithiasis: determination and prospective validation of a model predicting low risk. Am J Surg 1995; 170:38–43.

CLINICAL PREDICTION RULE

1. Patients were considered "low risk" if they met *all* four of the following criteria.
   - No jaundice
   - Normal transaminase levels
   - Common bile duct diameter <8 mm
   - No intrahepatic duct enlargement on conventional ultrasonography

Patients not meeting all of these criteria are "at risk" for common bile duct lithiasis.

2. The probability of CBDL is shown below for "low risk" and "at risk" patients in the prospective validation.

Risk group	No. of patients in this group	No. with CBDL	% With CBDL
At risk	108	42	39.0%
Low risk	168	1	0.6%

Note: Three low risk patients were lost to follow-up, and one low risk patient had a retained stone in the cystic duct.

Prognosis for Primary Biliary Cirrhosis

Clinical question

What is the prognosis for patients with primary biliary cirrhosis?

Population and setting

Patients at the Mayo Clinic with primary biliary cirrhosis who were enrolled in clinical trials of *d*-penicillamine were included. The mean age was 50 years; 12% were male; and 2% were of a nonwhite race. The validation group comprises patients who refused to participate in the trial. A total of 5% were histologic stage 1, 22% stage 2, 38% stage 3, and 35% stage 4. Patients were recruited between 1974 and 1984.

Study size

The training group had 312 patients and the validation group 106.

Pretest probability

Two years after the end of the enrollment period, 125 of the 312 patients in the training group had died after a median of 39 months in the study. Another 160 patients were still alive and being followed, with a median time in the study of 76 months; the rest were lost to follow-up ($n = 8$) or had undergone liver transplant ($n = 19$).

Type of validation

Grade II: The test set was a separate sample from the same population, with data for the test set gathered prospectively.

Comments

Although relatively old, treatment other than transplant has not advanced appreciably for biliary cirrhosis. This prediction model can give patients and their physicians an estimate of their prognosis. Because the model performed so well in the validation group, the model reported here is the result of a regression using all 418 patients.

Reference

Dickson ER, Grambsch PM, Fleming TR, et al. Prognosis in primary biliary cirrhosis: model for decision making. Hepatology 1989;10:1–7.

CLINICAL PREDICTION RULE

1. Calculate your patient's risk score R.

$$R = [0.871 \times \ln(\text{bilirubin in mg/dl})] - [2.53 \times \ln(\text{albumin in g/dl})] + [0.039 \times (\text{age in years})] + [2.38 \times \ln(\text{prothrombin time in seconds})] + [0.859 \times (\text{edema})]$$

Edema

0 = no edema and no diuretic therapy for edema

0.5 = edema present for which no diuretic therapy was given or edema resolved with diuretic therapy

1 = edema despite diuretic therapy

2. Find the value for S from the following table for the desired years of follow-up.

Years follow-up (n)	Prognosis at this many years (S)
1	0.97
2	0.941
3	0.883
4	0.833
5	0.774
6	0.721
7	0.651

3. Calculate the risk for this number of years.

$$\text{Probability of survival at n years} = S^{\exp(R-5.07)}$$

Example: Patient with total bilirubin 0.5 mg/dl, albumin 4.5 g/dl, age 52 years, PT 10.1 seconds, no edema, and no diuretics.

$$R = [0.871 \times \ln(0.5)] - [2.53 \times \ln(4.5)] + [0.039 \times 52] + [2.38 \times \ln(10.1)] + [0.859 \times 0.0] = 3.12$$

The estimated 5-year survival is $0.774^{\exp(3.12-5.07)} = 0.96$, so this patient has a 96% chance of surviving for 5 years.

4. The following table shows probabilities of survival for a range of R values.

	Probability of survival, by R score (from above)						
Years	0	2	4	6	8	10	>10
1	100%	100%	99%	93%	57%	1%	0%
2	100%	100%	98%	86%	32%	0%	0%
3	100%	99%	96%	73%	10%	0%	0%
4	100%	99%	94%	63%	3%	0%	0%
5	100%	99%	92%	52%	1%	0%	0%
6	100%	98%	89%	44%	0%	0%	0%
7	100%	98%	86%	34%	0%	0%	0%

Ranson's Criteria for Acute Pancreatitis Severity

Clinical question

What is the prognosis for patients with acute pancreatitis?

Population and setting

Consecutive patients in an Italian university hospital were included in a prospective validation study. The mean age was 61 years for those with severe disease and 58 years for those with mild disease.

Study size

Altogether, 91 patients were studied.

Pretest probability

Of these patients, 33% had severe disease.

Type of validation

Grade I: The test set was from a distinct population. The rule was developed in one group of patients and validated in another.

Comments

The study by deBernardinis et al. is one of the few prospective validations of the well known Ranson criteria. They showed that increasing scores are associated with increasing severity of disease and increasing mortality, in a fairly linear progression. The APACHE II score is another useful tool for prognosis in acute pancreatitis.

References

DeBernardinis M, Violi V, Roncoroni L, et al. Automated selection of high-risk patients with acute pancreatitis. Crit Care Med 1989;17:318–323.

Ranson JHC. Acute pancreatitis. Curr Probl Surg 1979;16:1–84.

CLINICAL PREDICTION RULE

1. Add up the number of risk factors for your patient.

Risk factor	Points
At admission or diagnosis	
Age > 70 years	1
White blood cell count > 18,000/mm^3	1
Blood glucose > 220 mg/dl	1
Serum LDH > 400 IU/L	1
Serum SGOT > 250 IU/L	1
During the initial 48 hours	
Hematocrit fall > 10%	1
BUN rise more than 2 mg/dl	1
Serum calcium < 8 mg/dl	1
Base deficit > 5 mEq/L	1
Fluid sequestration > 4000 ml	1
Total:	

2. The risk of severe disease and death is shown below.

Score	No. in group	Severe disease	Death
0	20	15%	5%
1	28	25%	14%
2	23	39%	22%
3	14	57%	43%
≥4	6	50%	50%

CT Severity Index for Acute Pancreatitis

Clinical question

What is the likelihood of death or serious morbidity in patients with acute pancreatitis, based on the results of a computed tomography (CT) scan?

Population and setting

Patients with acute pancreatitis admitted to a university medical center in New York were included. The mean age was 52 years (range 20–77 years), with 53 men and 35 women. The cause of pancreatitis was alcohol abuse in 30, cholelithiasis in 30, and unknown in 28.

Study size

Altogether, 88 patients were studied (training and validation group).

Pretest probability

The probability of death was 5.7%.

Type of validation

Grade IV: The training group was used as the validation group.

Comments

This clinical prediction rule, although fairly widely used, has never been prospectively validated. It should be used with caution and is included only because it is so widely described in the literature.

Reference

Balthazar EJ, Robinson DL, Megibow AJ, Ranson JH. Acute pancreatitis: value of CT in establishing prognosis. Radiology 1990;174:331–336.

CLINICAL PREDICTION RULE

1. Calculate your patient's CT severity index (range 0–10 points).

Risk factor	Points
Grade of acute pancreatitis by CT	
Normal pancreas	0
Pancreatic enlargement	1
Inflammation of pancreas and peripancreatic fat	2
One fluid collection or phlegmon	3
Two or more fluid collections or phlegmons	4
Degree of pancreatic necrosis by CT	
No necrosis	0
Necrosis of one-third of the pancreas	2
Necrosis of one-half of the pancreas	4
Necrosis of more than one-half of the pancreas	6
Total:	

2. The risk of mortality and complications is shown below.

CT severity index	Mortality	Complications
0–3	3%	8%
4–6	6%	35%
7–10	17%	92%

Note: Patients with a score of 0 or 1 had no mortality or complications. "Complications" was not clearly defined in the study, but probably referred to an abscess or pseudocyst. The number of patients in each risk group was not given.

8

Gynecology and Obstetrics

■ OBSTETRICS

Screening for Gestational Diabetes

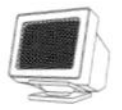

Clinical question

Is this patient at risk for gestational diabetes?

Population and setting

Pregnant women 24 years or older without known diabetes mellitus were recruited. All presented prior to 24 weeks' gestation to one of three Canadian teaching hospitals.

Study size

The training group had 1560 patients and the validation group 1571.

Pretest probability

Of these patients, 4% had gestational diabetes mellitus.

Type of validation

Grade II: The test set was a separate sample from the same population, with data for the test set gathered prospectively.

Comments

This was a large study with prospective validation. Although the standard of care is currently to screen all women for gestational diabetes, some are advocating a more selective approach, and this rule can give them a rational basis for their selection.

Reference

Naylor CD, Sermer M, Chen E, Farine D, for the Toronto Trihospital Gestational Diabetes Project Investigators. Selective screening for gestational diabetes mellitus. N Engl J Med 1997;337:1591–1596.

CLINICAL PREDICTION RULE

1. Calculate the body mass index (BMI).

$$\text{Weight (kg)} = \text{weight (pounds)}/2.2$$

$$\text{Height (m)} = \text{height (inches)} \times 0.0254$$

$$\text{BMI} = \text{weight (kg)}/\text{height (m)}^2$$

2. Count up your patient's risk factors.

Risk factor	Points
BMI	
0–22	0
>22–25	2
>25	3
Age (years)	
<31	0
31–34	1
>34	2
Race	
White	0
Black	0
Asian	5
Other	2
Total:	

3. Find the risk of gestational diabetes.

Risk score	No. of patients in this group	Probability of gestational diabetes mellitus
0–1	544	0.9%
2	322	3.7%
3	284	3.9%
4–5	330	7.3%
>5	91	18.7%

Probability of Successful Vaginal Birth after Cesarean Birth (Validated)

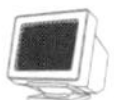

Clinical question

Which patients with a previous cesarean section will have a successful vaginal birth after a cesarean birth (VBAC)?

Population studied

The authors collected data on consecutive women in the Kaiser Permanente health system who had a trial of labor and a previous cesarean section. It was a diverse group of women: 38% were White, 37% Hispanic, 15% Black, and 10% from other ethnic groups. More than 95% were under age 40.

Study size

The training group had 2502 patients, and the score was validated in a group of 2501 patients.

Pretest probability

Altogether, 74.9% had a successful labor and delivered vaginally.

Type of validation

Grade II: The validation group was a separate sample from the same population, with data for the validation group gathered prospectively.

Comments

This is a well designed rule. The major limitation of the study design is the fact that data were abstracted from the medical record. However, the data elements should have been easily available in the record, and details of the data abstraction and training process of the abstractor are given.

Reference

Flamm BL, Geiger AM. Vaginal birth after cesarean delivery: an admission scoring system. Obstet Gynecol 1997;90:907–910.

CLINICAL PREDICTION RULE

1. Count up the number of points for your patient.

Patient characteristic	Points
Vaginal birth history	
Vaginal birth before and after first cesarean	4
Vaginal birth after first cesarean	2
Vaginal birth before first cesarean	1
No previous vaginal birth	0
Cervical effacement at admission	
>75%	2
25–75%	1
<25%	0
Cervical dilation 4 cm or more at admission	1
Reason other than failure to progress for first cesarean	1
Age under 40 years	2
Total:	

2. Find the likelihood of successful trial of labor in the table below.

Score	No. of women in validation group with this score	Probability of successful vaginal birth after cesarean section
0–2	114	49%
3	329	60%
4	595	67%
5	660	77%
6	350	89%
7	189	93%
8–10	158	95%

Probability of Successful Vaginal Birth after Cesarean Birth (Unvalidated)

Clinical question

Which patients with a previous cesarean section will have a successful vaginal birth after a cesarean birth (VBAC)?

Population studied

At an Israeli university hospital all patients with a previous cesarean section who underwent a trial of labor were included. Data were collected over a 10-year period; 4% were excluded because of lost records or insufficient data. The mean age was 32.5 years; the average parity was 3.4; and 38.9% had delivered vaginally before their cesarean section.

Study size

A total of 471 patients were studied.

Pretest probability

Of these patients, 78.1% had a successful trial of labor and delivered vaginally.

Type of validation

Grade IV: The training group was used as the validation group.

Comments

This is an otherwise well designed and potentially useful clinical rule, hampered by the lack of prospective validation. It should therefore be used with caution. Further prospective validation studies are needed.

Reference

Weinstein D, Benshushan A, Tanos V, Zilberstein R, Rojansky N. Predictive score for vaginal birth after cesarean section. Am J Obstet Gynecol 1996;174:192–198.

CLINICAL PREDICTION RULE

1. Count up the number of points for your patient.

Factor	Points
Bishop score ≥4	4
Vaginal delivery before cesarean section	2
Past indication (choose one primary indication only)	
Grade A (malpresentation, PIH, twins)	6
Grade B (placenta previa, abruptio placentae, prematurity, premature rupture of membranes)	5
Grade C (fetal distress, cephalopelvic disproportion or failure to progress, cord accident)	4
Grade D (macrosomia, IUGR)	3
Total:	

PIH = pregnancy-induced hypertension; IUGR = intrauterine growth retardation.

2. Find the likelihood of successful trial of labor in the table below.

Score	Probability of successful vaginal birth after cesarean section
≥4	≥58%
≥6	≥67%
≥8	≥78%
≥10	≥85%
≥12	≥88%

Successful Induction of Labor: Dhall Score

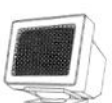

Clinical question

What is the likelihood of successful induction of labor?

Population and setting

Patients with a period of gestation from 36 to 43 weeks were included. In all cases, labor was induced for therapeutic reasons such as preeclampsia and hypertensive disorders ($n = 77$), postdates ($n = 51$), premature rupture of membranes ($n = 30$), and intrauterine growth retardation ($n = 11$). The attending physician was not aware of the patient's induction score. The method of induction varied: oxytocin infusion up to 16 mU/min in 189 patients (combined with amniotomy in 102) and amniotomy alone in 11 patients.

Study size

Altogether, 200 patients were studied.

Pretest probability

Labor was successful in 143 of 200 patients (71%).

Type of validation

Grade I: The validation group was from a distinct population. The rule was developed in one group of patients and validated in another.

Comments

This study prospectively compared the Dhall and Bishop scores. Because it was done by Dr. Dhall, one has to wonder whether he gave a subconscious boost to his namesake rule. However, the physicians doing the measurements were blinded to the scores, and the same measurements for effacement, dilatation, and consistency were used by both scores, reducing the risk of bias.

Reference

Dhall K, Mittal SC, Kumar A. Evaluation of preinduction scoring systems. Aust NZ J Obstet Gynaecol 1987;27:309–311.

CLINICAL PREDICTION RULE

1. Calculate your patient's Dhall score.

Variable	Points
Effacement	
0–30%	0
40–60%	1
>60%	2
Consistency	
Firm	0
Medium	2
Soft	4
Dilatation	
Closed	0
1–2 cm	3
3–4 cm	6
>4 cm	9
Parity	
Primipara	0
Multipara	4
Total (0–19):	

2. The duration of induction and the likelihood of successful induction of labor is shown below.

Dhall score	Mean induction to delivery interval	Success rate
0–6	21.1 hours	34%
7–8	15.8 hours	72%
>8	10.8 hours	91%

3. Results are shown in more detail below.

Dhall score	Success rate
0–1	0%
2–4	25%
5	35%
6	42%
7	62%
8	76%
9	86%
10–12	90%
13–19	95%

Successful Induction of Labor: Bishop Score

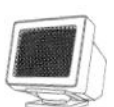

Clinical question

What is the likelihood of successful induction of labor?

Population and setting

Patients with a period of gestation from 36 to 43 weeks were included. In all cases, labor was induced for therapeutic reasons such as preeclampsia and hypertensive disorders (n = 77), postdates (n = 51), premature rupture of membranes (n = 30), and intrauterine growth retardation (n = 11). The attending physician was not aware of the patient's induction score. The method of induction varied; with oxytocin infusion up to 16 mU/min in 189 patients (combined with amniotomy in 102) and amniotomy alone in 11 patients.

Study size

Altogether, 200 patients were studied.

Pretest probability

Labor was successful in 143 of 200 patients (71%).

Type of validation

Grade I: The validation group was from a distinct population. The rule was developed in one group of patients and validated in another.

Comments

This study prospectively compared the Dhall and Bishop scores. Because the first author was Dr. Dhall, one has to wonder whether he gave a subconscious boost to his namesake's clinical rule. However, the physicians doing the measurements were blinded to the scores; and the same measurements for effacement, dilatation, and consistency were used by both scores, reducing the risk of bias.

Reference

Dhall K, Mittal SC, Kumar A. Evaluation of preinduction scoring systems. Aust NZ J Obstet Gynaecol 1987;27:309–311.

CLINICAL PREDICTION RULE

1. Calculate your patient's Bishop score.

Variable	Points
Effacement	
0–30%	0
40–50%	1
60–70%	2
80%–100%	3
Consistency	
Firm	0
Medium	1
Soft	2
Dilatation	
Closed	0
1–2 cm	1
3–4 cm	2
≥5 cm	3
Position	
Posterior	0
Middle	1
Anterior	2
Station	
−3	0
−2	1
−1 or 0	2
+1 or +2	3
Total (0–13):	

2. The duration of induction and the likelihood of successful induction of labor is shown below:

Bishop score	Mean induction to delivery interval	Success rate
0–3	19.4 hours	47%
4–5	15.9 hours	68%
>5	9.4 hours	92%

3. Results are shown in more detail below.

Bishop score	Success rate
0–2	42%
3	54%
4	73%
5	61%
6	90%
7–8	94%

Predicting Success of External Cephalic Version

Clinical question

What is the likelihood of success of external cephalic version of a breech presentation?

Population and setting

Women with a singleton gestation with a breech presentation undergoing external cephalic version were included. Women were excluded for abruptio placentae, placenta previa, premature rupture of membranes, or evidence of fetal compromise during preliminary fetal heart rate monitoring.

Study size

The training group had 108 patients and the validation group 266.

Pretest probability

External cephalic version was successful 62.4% of the time and was performed at a mean gestational age of 37.8 weeks.

Type of validation

Grade II: The validation group was a separate sample from the same population, with data for the validation group gathered prospectively.

Comments

The protocol used was as follows: After a reactive nonstress test or negative contraction stress test, either ritodrine hydrochloride at 100 μg/min or terbutaline sulfate at 250 μg SC was given. After 20 minutes external version was attempted by two physicians. The "forward roll" technique was usually attempted if the fetal head crossed the maternal midline. The "back flip" was used if the initial method failed or, occasionally, as the initial technique if the fetus did not cross the midline. Attempts were stopped if there was patient discomfort or abnormal fetal heart tracings, or after multiple failed attempts.

Reference

Newman RB, Peacock BS, VanDorsten JP, Hunt HH. Predicting success of external cephalic version. Am J Obstet Gynecol 1993;169:245–250.

CLINICAL PREDICTION RULE

1. Calculate the patient's external cephalic version score (range 0–10).

Risk factor	Points
Parity	
0	0
1	1
≥2	2
Dilatation (cm)	
≥3	0
1–2	1
0	2
Estimated weight (g)	
<2500 g	0
2500–3500 g	1
>3500 g	2
Placenta	
Anterior	0
Posterior	1
Lateral/fundal	2
Station	
≥ −1	0
−2	1
≤ −3	2
Total:	

2. The percent success of external cephalic version for a given score is shown below.

Score	No. of women	Successful external cephalic version
0–2	13	0%
3–4	30	33%
5–7	174	65%
8	30	80%
9–10	19	100%

9

Hematology/Oncology

THYROID CANCER

Thyroid Carcinoma Prognosis

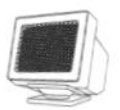

Clinical question

What is the prognosis for patients with thyroid carcinoma?

Population studied

Patients were drawn from a European Thyroid Cancer Registry. Those with incomplete information or lost to follow-up were excluded (n = 84). The median age was 50 years; 68% were female.

Study size

Altogether, 507 patients were studied.

Pretest probability

The 5-year survival rate was 64% for all patients.

Type of validation

Grade IV: The training group was used as the validation group.

Comments

This rule should be used with caution because it has not been prospectively validated. Otherwise, the variables used are clear and unambiguous, and the size of the population is adequate.

Reference

Byar DP, Green SB, Dor P, et al. A prognostic index for thyroid carcinoma: a study of the EORTC Thyroid Cancer Cooperative Group. Eur J Cancer 1979;15:1033–1041.

CLINICAL PREDICTION RULE

1. Add up the number of points for your patient, including the number of years as one variable (e.g., a 40-year-old male patient with an anaplastic tumor and one distant metastatic site would have 40 + 12 + 45 + 15 = 112 points).

Variable	Points
Age at diagnosis (years)	(years)
Male gender	12
If medullary *or* if principal cell type is follicular less differentiated, provided the associated cell type is not anaplastic	10
If principal or associated cell type is anaplastic	45
If T category is T3	15
If there is at least one distant metastatic site	15
In addition to above, if there are multiple distant metastatic sites	15
Total:	

2. Observed 5-year survival by risk group is as follows.

Score	Risk group	Observed 5-year survival
<50	1	95%
50–65	2	80%
66–83	3	51%
84–108	4	33%
≥109	5	5%

FUNCTION/PERFORMANCE SCALES

Karnofsky Performance Scale

Clinical question

How long will this terminally ill patient live?

Population and setting

This was a population of adult patients with a biopsy-confirmed diagnosis of cancer (unless brain or pancreatic in which case computed tomography (CT) scan could be used to confirm the diagnosis). All patients were being evaluated for entry into a hospice program, and only patients with a Karnofsky Performance Scale score of ≤ 50 ("requires considerable assistance from others and frequent medical care") were included.

Study size

Altogether, 685 patients were studied.

Pretest probability

This parameter is not applicable.

Type of validation

Grade I: The test set was from a distinct population. The rule was developed in one group of patients and validated in another.

Comments

It is important to understand and appreciate that although the Karnofsky Performance Scale is, on average, quite accurate for populations the variation in actual outcomes for individuals can be quite large. For example, a score of 20–30 in an Italian study was associated with survival of as little as 1 week and as much as 12 weeks, and a score of 40–50 was associated with survival of as little as 1 week and as much as 24 weeks.

Reference

Mor V, Laliberte L, Morris JN, Wiemann M. The Karnofsky Performance Status Scale: an examination of its reliability and validity in a research setting. Cancer 1984;53:2002–2007.

CLINICAL PREDICTION RULE

1. Calculate the Karnofsky score.

Definition	Criteria
Able to carry on normal activity and to work. No special care is needed.	
100%	Normal; no complaints; no evidence of disease
90%	Able to carry on normal activity; minor signs or symptoms of disease
80%	Normal activity with effort; some signs or symptoms of disease
Unable to work. Able to live at home, care for most personal needs. A varying amount of assistance is needed.	
70%	Cares for self; unable to carry on normal activity or to do active work
60%	Requires occasional assistance but is able to care for most of his or her needs
50%	Requires considerable assistance from others and frequent medical care
Unable to care for self. Requires equivalent of institutional or hospital care. Disease may be progressing rapidly.	
40%	Disabled; requires special care and assistance
30%	Severely disabled; hospitalization is indicated although death not imminent
20%	Very sick; hospitalization necessary; active support treatment necessary
10%	Moribund; fatal processes progressing rapidly
0%	Dead

2. The estimated longevity is shown below. The scale is not a good predictor of longevity for scores > 50. Note also the large standard deviation; there is considerable variability in survival within each level of the Karnofsky Performance Scale (KPS).

KPS index	No. of patients with this score	Mean longevity (days) (SD)	Median longevity (days)
10	13	17.6 (20.5)	9.5
20	84	27.1 (29.4)	17.8
30	239	45.7 (43.4)	31.9
40	244	64.1 (52.4)	46.7
50	105	72.0 (52.8)	59.7

3. Another way to look at this information is shown below for the same set of patients. The values shown are the percentage of patients receiving each score who survive for the number of days shown. For example, 21.4% of patients with a score of 10 survive 19–36 days, and 7.1% survive for at least 37 days.

	Patients with KPS scores of 10–50				
Patient longevity (days)	10	20	30	40	50
1–18	71.4%	52.2%	29.1%	13.9%	8.7%
19–36	21.4%	25.0%	27.6%	26.6%	20.9%
≥37	7.1%	22.6%	43.3%	59.6%	70.4%

LUNG CANCER

Prognosis for Inoperable Non-Small-Cell Lung Cancer

Clinical question

What is the likelihood of survival to 3 months for patients with inoperable non-small-cell lung cancer?

Population and setting

Patients were included if they had inoperable non-small-cell lung cancer, had had no previous radiotherapy or chemotherapy, and were referred for palliative radiotherapy. The mean age was 63 years; 79 of 96 patients in the training group were women.

Study size

The training group had 96 patients and the validation group 80.

Pretest probability

Of patients in the validation group, 24% died before 3 months.

Type of validation

Grade II: The validation group was a separate sample from the same population, with data for the validation group gathered prospectively.

Comments

This prospectively validated prognostic index can help determine an appropriate radiation dose for patients with inoperable non-small-cell lung cancer given their likelihood of surviving more than 3 months.

Reference

Thorogood J, Bulman AS, Collins T, Ash D. The use of discriminant analysis to guide palliative treatment for lung cancer patients. Clin Oncol 1992;4:22–36.

CLINICAL PREDICTION RULE

1. Count up the number of risk factors for your patient.

Risk factor	Points
More than 10 lb weight loss	1
WHO performance status of 3 or 4	1
Extensive disease (versus limited disease)	1
Lymphocyte count $\leq 1 \times 10^9$/L	1
Total:	

2. Determine their likelihood of survival to 3 months.

No. of points	Probability of survival to 3 months
0 or 1	$\geq$ 95%
2	60–74%
3 or 4	< 20%

Prognosis for Terminal Lung Cancer

Clinical question

What is the prognosis for patients with terminal lung cancer?

Population and setting

Consecutive lung cancer patients admitted to a community-based, nonprofit home hospice service were studied. The mean age was 68 years; 25% were over age 75; 65% were male.

Study size

There were 310 patients in the training group and 78 in the validation group.

Pretest probability

The mean survival was 51 days; median survival was 27 days.

Type of validation

Grade II: The validation group was a separate sample from the same population, with data for the validation group gathered prospectively.

Comments

Unfortunately, most patients are referred to a hospice too late to benefit fully from the services. This well designed and tested clinical rule can help identify patients with a poor prognosis who should be referred.

Reference

Schonwetter RS, Robinson BE, Ramirez G. Prognostic factors for survival in terminal lung cancer patients. J Gen Intern Med 1994;9:366–371.

CLINICAL PREDICTION RULE

1. Count the number of the following characteristics your patient has.

Characteristic	Points
Pulse (tachycardic)	1
Toileting (needs assistance or dependent)	1
Feeding (needs assistance or dependent)	1
Absence of a living will	1
Tissue type (other than adenocarcinoma or squamous cell cancer)	1
Dry mouth	1
Liver metastasis	1
Pain (severe or incapacitating)	1
Total:	

2. Find the estimated duration of survival based on the number of characteristics.

Score	No.	50% Mortality (days)	90% Mortality (days)
1	4	83	443
2	26	71	346
3	42	46	184
4	78	37	121
5	65	19	67
6	58	9	65
7	26	9	34
8	6	3	10

Prognosis for Inoperable Bronchogenic Lung Cancer

Clinical question

What is the prognosis for patients with inoperable bronchogenic carcinoma of the lung?

Population and setting

Patients of the Veteran's Administration Lung Group with inoperable bronchogenic lung cancer treated with one of six experimental protocols during the 1960s and 1970s were included; almost all were male.

Study size

A total of 5138 patients were studied.

Pretest probability

Of the 5138 patients, 4840 (94%) were known to have died.

Type of validation

Grade IV: The training group was used as the validation group.

Comments

The obvious limitation is the age of this study, with data largely collected during the 1960s and 1970s. On the other hand, the prognosis for patients with inoperable lung cancer has not changed dramatically since that time. The estimates are probably slightly low, though, given that there has been some improvement in care. Prospective validation is needed.

Reference

Stanley KE. Prognostic factors for survival in patients with inoperable lung cancer. J Natl Cancer Inst 1980;65:25–32.

CLINICAL PREDICTION RULE

1. Determine the patient's Karnofsky Performance Score (see page 179).
2. Determine the patient's estimated median survival.

	Length of survival (weeks)								
				Disease extending beyond one hemithorax					
	Disease confined to one hemithorax			No scalene or supraclavicular nodal involvement			Scalene and/or supraclavicular nodal involvement		
Initial Karnofsky Score	No wt loss	Wt loss <10%	Wt loss >10%	No Wt loss	Wt loss <10%	Wt loss >10%	No Wt loss	Wt loss <10%	Wt loss >10%
100	72	54	43	41	31	26	33	26	21
90	55	41	33	32	25	20	26	20	17
80	48	36	30	29	22	18	23	18	15
70	42	32	27	26	20	16	21	16	13
60	33	26	21	20	16	13	16	13	10
50	26	20	17	16	12	10	13	10	8
40	21	16	13	13	10	8	10	7	6

BREAST CANCER

Risk of Breast Cancer (Gail Risk Model)

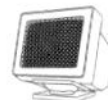

Clinical question

What is a woman's risk of developing breast cancer over the next 10, 20, or 30 years?

Population and setting

Women who were part of the Breast Cancer Detection Demonstration Project were included. This included both patients who had a breast cancer between 1973 and 1980 and controls who did not. Only data from white women were used to develop the rule.

Study size

The rule was developed from 2852 cases and 3146 controls.

Pretest probability

Because this was a case–control design the pretest probability is not applicable.

Type of validation

Grade IV: The training group was used as the validation group.

Comments

This widely used clinical rule helps determine the 10-year risk of breast cancer. The 20-year and 30-year risks are calculable for young women. Prospective validation is needed and will probably be available by the time of publication of the next edition of this manual.

Reference

Gail MH, Brinton LA, Byar DP, et al. Projecting individualized probabilities of developing breast cancer for white females who are being examined annually. J Natl Cancer Inst 1989;81:1879–1886.

CLINICAL PREDICTION RULE

1. First, estimate your patient's initial relative risk of breast cancer based on her risk factors. Write the relative risk for each of the three risk factor combinations in the final column next to A, B, and C. Then, multiply A × B × C for the patients overall relative risk.

Risk factor	No. of first-degree relatives with breast cancer[a]	Associated relative risk	Total relative risk
Age at menarche (years)			
≥14	NA	1.000	
12–13	NA	1.099	
<12	NA	1.207	*A*:
No. of previous breast biopsies			
Age <50 years			
0	NA	1.000	
1	NA	1.698	
>1	NA	2.882	
Age ≥50 years			
0	NA	1.000	
1	NA	1.273	
>1	NA	1.620	*B*:
Age at first live birth (years)			
<20	0	1.000	
<20	1	2.607	
<20	>1	6.798	
20–24	0	1.244	
20–24	1	2.681	
20–24	>1	5.750	
25–29 or nulliparous	0	1.548	
25–29 or nulliparous	1	2.756	
25–29 or nulliparous	>1	4.907	
>29	0	1.927	
>29	1	2.834	
>29	>1	4.169	*C*:
		A × B × C	

[a]Mother or sisters.

2. Find your patient's initial age and desired years of follow-up in the first two columns. If the initial age plus the years of follow-up is more than 50, you have to also specify a "later relative risk." This is done using part 1 above but substituting values for the woman at the end of follow-up. For example, if the patient is 40 years old and you want to estimate the risk of breast cancer over the next 30 years, calculate her "initial relative risk" using age 40 and her risk factors and the "later relative risk" using age 70 and her current risk factors.

Initial age (years)	Years of follow-up	Later relative risk	Initial relative risk[a]					
			1.0	2.0	5.0	10.0	20.0	30.0
20	10		0	0.1	0.2	0.5	1.0	1.4
	20		0.5	1.0	2.5	4.9	9.5	14.0
	30		1.7	3.4	8.3	15.9	29.3	40.5
30	10		0.5	0.9	2.3	4.4	8.7	12.8
	20		1.7	3.3	8.1	15.6	28.8	39.9
	30	1.0	3.2	4.8	9.5	16.9	29.9	40.8
		2.0	4.7	6.3	10.9	18.2	30.9	41.7
		5.0	8.9	10.4	14.9	21.8	34.0	44.3
		10.0	15.6	17.1	21.2	27.6	38.8	48.3
		20.0	27.6	28.8	32.3	37.8	47.4	55.5
		30.0	37.7	38.7	41.8	46.4	54.7	61.7
40	10		1.2	2.5	6.1	11.8	22.2	31.3
	20	1.0	2.8	4.0	7.5	13.1	23.4	32.4
		2.0	4.3	5.5	8.9	14.5	24.5	33.4
		5.0	8.6	9.7	13.1	18.3	28.0	36.4
		10.0	15.4	16.4	19.5	24.4	33.3	41.1
		20.0	24.0	28.4	30.9	35.2	42.7	49.5
		30.0	37.7	38.5	40.7	44.3	50.8	56.6
	30	1.0	4.4	5.6	9.1	14.6	24.6	33.5
		2.0	7.4	8.6	11.9	17.3	27.0	35.6
		5.0	15.9	17.0	20.0	24.9	33.7	41.5
		10.0	28.3	29.2	31.8	35.9	43.4	50.0
		20.0	47.5	48.1	50.0	53.1	58.5	63.4
		30.0	61.2	61.6	63.1	65.3	69.3	72.8
50	10		1.6	3.1	7.6	14.6	27.1	37.7
	20		3.2	6.4	15.1	27.9	47.8	61.9
	30		4.4	8.5	19.9	35.5	57.8	71.7
60	10		1.8	3.6	8.6	16.5	30.1	41.5
	20		3.0	5.9	14.0	25.9	44.6	58.2
70	10		1.4	2.7	6.7	12.9	24.1	33.7

[a]Percent probability of breast cancer over the years of follow-up.

Example: What is the 20 year risk for a 40-year-old woman with menarche at age 13 ($A = 1.099$), one previous breast biopsy ($B = 1.698$), first live birth at age 22, and a mother with breast cancer ($C = 2.681$). The product of A, B, and C for the calculation of "initial relative risk" is $1.099 \times 1.698 \times 2.681 = 5.00$. The "later relative risk" is calculated the same way, although the value for B is now 1.273 because we are looking at her risk at age 60 (initial 40 + 20 years). The "later relative risk" is therefore $1.099 \times 1.273 \times 2.681 = 3.75$. To find her risk of breast cancer for the next 20 years, go down the first column to age 40, then down one more row to a 20-year risk estimate. Because the "later relative risk" is 3.75, look at both the 2.0 and 5.0 rows and interpolate. Go across to the "initial relative risk" estimate of 5.0, and you see that for a "later relative risk" of 2.0 the patient's risk is 8.9%, and for the "later relative risk" of 5.0 it is 13.1%. You interpolate in your head and estimate an 11% risk of breast cancer over the next 20 years for your patient.

Risk of Breast Cancer Recurrence after Simple Mastectomy

Clinical question

What is the likelihood of local recurrence after simple mastectomy?

Population and setting

Women who underwent a simple mastectomy for invasive primary operable breast cancer measuring less than 5 cm were included. The mean age was 58 years, and patients were excluded if they were over 70 years old.

Study size

A total of 966 patients were studied.

Pretest probability

Of these patients, 23% had a local recurrence.

Type of validation

Grade IV: The training group was used as the validation group.

Comments

This large study is limited by the lack of detailed information on participants and the failure to validate the clinical rule prospectively. It should therefore be used with caution. It was otherwise well designed, though, and has adequate sample size.

Reference

O'Rourke S, Galea MH, Morgan D, et al. Local recurrence after simple mastectomy. Br J Surg 1994;81:386–389.

CLINICAL PREDICTION RULE

1. Add up the points for your patient.

Variable	Points
Tumor grade	
I	6
II	12
III	18
Lymph node status	
Negative	6
Positive	12
Lymphovascular invasion	
Absent	4
Present	8
Total:	

2. The likelihood of local recurrence for each possible score is shown below.

Score	Patients with this score	Local recurrence with this score
16	11%	8.5%
20	1%	12.5%
22	20%	15.8%
26	6%	10.0%
28	29%	15.5%
32	13%	33.0%
34	9%	38.5%
38	11%	48.0%
All Patients	100%	23.0%

Prognosis in Metastatic Breast Cancer

Clinical question

What is the prognosis for patients with metastatic breast cancer?

Population and setting

This Japanese study used a group of patients who were part of a trial to compare tamoxifen versus medroxyprogesterone acetate in combination with doxorubicin and cyclophosphamide for metastatic breast cancer. Patients were accrued between 1988 and 1991 and followed for a median of 25 months; the median follow-up for those still alive was 79.9 months. The validation group consisted of patients treated with standard anthracycline-containing regimens at the Japanese National Cancer Center Hospital. The authors admit that the validation group may be a more highly selected group. In the training group, 29% were under age 50.

Study size

The training group had 218 patients and the validation group 279.

Pretest probability

The mean survival in the validation group was 28.0 months; the 5-year survival rate was 22.5%.

Type of validation

Grade I: The test set was from a distinct population. The rule was developed in one group of patients and validated in another.

Comments

The major limitation of this rule for physicians in the United States and Europe is the question of generalizability from a Japanese population. Note that receiving adjuvant chemotherapy decreased the mean survival time, which seems counterintuitive. This may represent a selection bias (i.e., patients selected to receive adjuvant therapy had a worse prognosis), or it may represent worse outcomes due to the morbidity associated with the adjuvant therapy.

Reference

Yamamoto N, Watanabe T, Katsumata N, et al. Construction and validation of a practical prognostic index for patients with metastatic breast cancer. J Clin Oncol 1998;16:2401–2408.

CLINICAL PREDICTION RULE

1. Calculate the patient's risk score.

Risk factor	Points
Received adjuvant chemotherapy after surgery	1
Presents with distant lymph node metastasis	1
Presents with liver metastasis	1
Serum LDH > upper limit of normal	1
Disease-free interval < 24 months	2
Total:	

2. Estimate the patient's mean survival time.

Risk score	No. of patients	Mean survival (months)	1-Year survival	3-Year survival	5-Year survival
≤1	97	49.6	96%	76%	36%
2–3	93	22.8	80%	47%	14%
≥4	44	10.0	41%	10%	0%

Long-term Outcome for Breast Cancer

Clinical question

What is the long-term outcome for patients with breast cancer?

Population studied

Women with primary breast cancer treated at a Finnish university hospital for whom complete follow-up data were available (we do not know how many were excluded). The mean age was 59 years; 50% were axillary node-positive; and the mean duration of follow-up was 12.5 years. Modified mastectomy was the treatment for 285 patients, mastectomy plus adjuvant therapy for 320, hormone therapy for 81, and no treatment for 6.

Study size

The validation group had 609 patients.

Pretest probability

The likelihood of being recurrence-free during the follow-up period was 55%. There were 290 survivors (47.6%), 275 died of breast cancer (45.1%), and 88 died of other causes (14.4%).

Type of validation

Grade I: The validation group was from a distinct population. The rule was developed in one group of patients and validated in another.

Comments

This clinical rule uses morphometric data to assist in prognostication, which may not be readily available to primary care physicians or surgeons at your institution. Different cutoffs are reported for the interpretation of the rule. This rule is most useful to pathologists.

Reference

Aaltomaa S, Lipponen P, Eskelinen M, et al. Predictive value of a morphometric prognostic index in female breast cancer. Oncology 1993;50:57–62.

CLINICAL PREDICTION RULE

Definitions

MAl = mitotic activity index: number of mitotic figures in 10 consecutive fields with an objective magnification of ×40 (field diameter 490 μm)

MPI = morphometric predictive index

pN = 1 if axillary node positive, 2 if auxiliary node negative

$$\text{MPI} = (0.3341 \times \sqrt{\text{MAI}}) + (0.2342 \times \text{tumor size in cm}) - (0.7654 \times pN)$$

Parameter	All patients	Axillary node-negative patients	Axillary node-positive patients
Patients recurrence-free at a mean follow-up of 12.5 years			
MPI ≤ 0	**75%**	75%	50%
MPI > 0	**50%**	60%	45%
MPI ≤ 0.6	65%	70%	**55%**
MPI > 0.6	50%	55%	**45%**
MAI ≤ 10	60%	**75%**	50%
MAI > 10	50%	**55%**	45%
Patients alive at a mean follow-up of 12.5 years			
MPI ≤ 0	75	75	**100**
MPI > 0	40	60	**30**
MPI ≤ 0.6	**70**	**75**	55
MPI > 0.6	**35**	**55**	25
MAI ≤ 10	60	75	35
MAI > 10	40	60	25

Note: the predictor with the best ability to discriminate is highlighted in boldface for each patient outcome.

HEPATOCELLULAR CARCINOMA

Risk of Hepatocellular Carcinoma with Cirrhosis

Clinical question

What is the risk of developing hepatocellular carcinoma (HCC) among patients with cirrhosis?

Population and setting

Consecutive patients hospitalized between 1987 and 1990 in a French teaching hospital who had cirrhosis but no detectable HCC were included. Diagnosis was based on ultrasonography and serum α-fetoprotein (AFP) < 250 ng/ml. The training group included 85 men and 66 women. Cirrhosis was caused by alcohol use in 71, hepatitis C virus (HCV) in 28, alcohol plus HCV in 22, hemochromatosis in 7, primary biliary cirrhosis in 7, hepatitis B in 6, autoimmunity in 5, and unknown cause in 5. The validation group included 27 men and 22 women. Cirrhosis was caused by alcohol use in 33, HCV in 6, alcohol plus HCV in 6, hemochromatosis in 3, and primary biliary cirrhosis in 1. The mean age of both groups was 57 years.

Study size

The training group had 151 patients and the validation group 49.

Pretest probability

Of the 151 patients, 31 (20%) developed HCC in the training group during the 4 to 7-year follow-up.

Type of validation

Grade II: Clinical rule was developed using one group of patients and was tested prospectively using a second group of patients at the same institution.

Comments

Patients at higher risk for HCC could perhaps be screened more aggressively with ultrasonography and serum AFP, although there is no evidence that doing so would necessarily improve clinical outcomes.

Reference

Ganne-Carrie N, Chastang C, Chapel F, et al. Predictive score for the development of hepatocellular carcinoma and additional value of liver large cell dysplasia in Western patients with cirrhosis. Hepatology 1996;23:1112–1118.

CLINICAL PREDICTION RULE

1. Count up the points for your patient.

Risk factor	Points
Age ≥ 50 years	6
Male gender	4
Large esophageal varices (grade II or III)	3
Prothrombin activity < 70%	3
Serum AFP ≥ 15 ng/L	3
Anti-HCV antibodies present	3
Total (0–22):	

2. Determine your patient's risk of developing HCC at 3 years.

Points	Risk of HCC in training group	Risk of HCC in validation group
< 11	0% (0–3%)	6% (0–18%)
≥ 11	24% (14–34%)	44% (22–66%)

Numbers in parentheses are the 95% confidence interval.

OVARIAN CANCER

Ovarian Cancer Prognosis

Clinical question

Which patients with stage III or IV ovarian carcinoma and no evidence of disease after surgery and chemotherapy will be cured (median follow-up 42 months)?

Population and setting

Patients entered in a National Cancer Institute of Canada trial at multiple centers were studied. Only patients with stage III or IV ovarian carcinoma and no evidence of disease after surgery and chemotherapy (adriamycin and cisplatin) who underwent second-look laparotomy were included. Most ($n = 146$) were stage III. The performance status was 0 for 62 patients, 1 for 62, 2 for 20, and 3 for 2.

Study size

Altogether, 173 patients were studied.

Pretest probability

Of these patients, 13.3% were cured, with a median follow-up of 42 months.

Type of validation

Grade IV: The training group was used as the validation group.

Comments

This rule gives us some prognostic information for patients with advanced ovarian carcinoma who appear to have no evidence of disease after treatment, although most still do badly. Also, this rule has not been prospectively validated and should therefore be used with caution.

Reference

Carmichael JA, Shelley WE, Brown LB, et al. A predictive index of cure versus no cure in advanced ovarian carcinoma patients: replacement of second-look laparotomy as a diagnostic test. Gynecol Oncol 1987;27:269–278.

CLINICAL PREDICTION RULE

1. Patients with at least two of the following three characteristics were in the poor prognosis group (the remainder were in the good performance group).
   - Age > 60 years
   - Macroscopic residual initially
   - Performance status 2 or 3 initially

2. The probability of cure for poor and good performance groups are shown below.

Parameter	Poor performance group	Good performance group
Negative second look	23%	39%
Negative second look, with relapse	91%	34%
All patients	2.2%	25%

HEMATOLOGIC TUMORS

Multiple Myeloma

Clinical question

What is the prognosis for patients with multiple myeloma?

Population and setting

Patients enrolled in an Italian randomized multicenter trial were included. Detailed demographic information is not given. The mean duration of follow-up was 42 months.

Study size

Altogether, 231 patients were studied.

Pretest probability

This parameter is not applicable.

Type of validation

Grade IV: The training group was used as the validation group.

Comments

This clinical rule was developed from patients enrolled in Italian treatment trials. Patients treated differently may have a different prognosis, although the difference in outcome between treatment groups was small in this study. Note that this clinical rule was not prospectively validated and should therefore be used with caution.

Reference

Grignani G, Gobbi PG, Formisano R, et al. A prognostic index for multiple myeloma. Br J Cancer 1996;73:1101–1107.

CLINICAL PREDICTION RULE

1. Calculate the patient's total score.

Variable	Points
British Medical Research Council Stage	
I	0.5
II	1.0
III	1.5
Bone marrow infiltrate cytology[a]	
BMI and BMC both favorable	0.5
BMI or BMC unfavorable	1.0
BMI and BMC both unfavorable	1.5
Treatment response at 6 months[b]	
Complete	0
Partial	1.5
No response	3.0
Total:	

[a]BMI = bone marrow plasma cell percentage; BMC = bone marrow plasma cell cytologic feature (plasma cell vs. plasmablast).

[b]Therapeutic response considered the following six criteria.

1. Reduction in the monoclonal component
2. Decrease in bone marrow plasma cells of at least 20% or a return to less than 20% as evaluated on bone marrow imprints before and after treatment
3. A ≥ 2 g/dl rise in hemoglobin (Hb) concentration in anemic patients (Hb < 11 g/dl) sustained for > 4 months
4. Return of serum calcium and BUN to normal values
5. Elevation of serum albumin to 3 g/dl or higher in the absence of other causes of hypoalbuminemia
6. Absence of progression of skeletal lytic lesions

Complete response = > 50% reduction in the monoclonal component and a response in at least three of the other five criteria

Partial response = 25–50% reduction in the monoclonal component and a response in at least three of the other five criteria

No response = failure to fulfill the above criteria for partial or complete response

2. Interpret the score using this table.

Risk class	Score	Median survival	Death rate (%)
I	0–1	52 months	59%
II	2	28 months	82%
III	3–5	13 months	98%

ALL MALIGNANCIES

Fever and Neutropenia in Cancer Patients

Clinical question

Which cancer patients with fever and neutropenia are at risk for serious medical complications?

Population and setting

Consecutive cancer patients with fever (temperature > 100.5°F) and neutropenia (granulocyte count < 500/μl) were recruited. Patients came from a cancer center (n = 383) and a general medical service (n = 61). The median age was 44 years (range 18–81 years); 53% were male; 24% had non-Hodgkin's lymphoma, 17% acute myelogenous leukemia, 12% breast cancer, and 47% another malignancy.

Study size

The validation group had 444 patients.

Pretest probability

Of these patients, 27% had a serious medical complication; 8% died.

Type of validation

Grade I: The validation group was from a distinct population. The rule was developed in one group of patients and validated in another.

Comments

This is a well designed rule with a thorough, independent validation in a large group of hospitalized patients. It can help clinicians identify patients who are at a particularly high risk of complications and so require special monitoring.

Reference

Talcott JA, Siegel RD, Finberg R, Goldman L. Risk assessment in cancer patients with fever and neutropenia: a prospective, two-center validation of a prediction rule. J Clin Oncol 1992;10:316–322.

CLINICAL PREDICTION RULE

1. Review the following definitions.
   Serious co-morbidities: Any condition other than fever and neutropenia that independently required inpatient observation or therapy. Predefined co-morbidities: hypotension (systolic blood pressure < 90 mm Hg), altered mental status, respiratory failure (PO_2 < 60 mm Hg), uncontrolled bleeding with platelet count < 40,000/μl, inadequate outpatient fluid intake or pain control, suspected spinal cord compression, and symptomatic hypercalcemia. Other co-morbidities: need for induction therapy, serious localized infection, acute abdomen, new deep vein thrombosis, witnessed syncopal episode, obstructed J tube, symptomatic, suspected perirectal abscess, and combination of hyperglycemia, severe anemia, and profound weakness.
   Uncontrolled cancer: For leukemia: absence of documented complete remission. For lymphoma or solid tumors: development of new lesions, 25% or more enlargement of a measurable lesion while on chemotherapy, or premature termination of chemotherapy due to other evidence of failure. Patients with evidence of disease progression when not receiving active systemic therapy were rated as not having uncontrolled cancer.
2. The risk of complications or mortality is shown below.

Risk Group	Description	No. of patients in this group	Serious medical complications	Mortality
I	Inpatients	268	35%	9%
II	Outpatients who demonstrated serious concurrent co-morbidity within 24 hours of presentation	43	33%	12%
III	Outpatients without serious concurrent co-morbidity but with uncontrolled cancer	29	21%	14%
IV	All other patients (outpatients without serious co-morbidity or uncontrolled cancer)	104	5%	0%

DERMATOLOGIC MALIGNANCIES

Prognosis for Melanoma

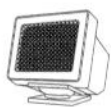

Clinical question

What is the prognosis in terms of 10-year survival for patients with melanoma?

Population and setting

Patients evaluated at a university medical center for primary melanoma between 1972 and 1979 were included. Exclusion criteria included: death during follow-up ($n = 44$), lack of follow-up ($n = 22$), metastatic disease at presentation ($n = 29$), inadequate surgical treatment ($n = 14$), and other ($n = 27$). The median age was 48 years; 54% were female.

Study size

The training group had 488 patients and the validation group 142.

Pretest probability

The 10-year survival rate was 78%, with 104 of 488 patients dying before 10 years. The median duration of follow-up was 13.5 years.

Type of validation

Grade II: The validation group was a separate sample from the same population, with data for the validation group gathered prospectively.

Comments

This was a well designed study, with a long duration of follow-up and adequate validation. It provides accurate prognostic estimates for patients with a newly diagnosed melanoma. It was also independently validated by Margolis and colleagues in a different population for prediction of 5-year prognosis. Of the four factors, thickness is by far the most important, and Margolis found that thickness alone was almost as good a predictor of survival as the entire model.

References

Margolis DJ, Halpeen AC, Rebbeck T, et al. Validation of a melanoma prognostic model. Arch Dermatol 1998;134:1597–1601.

Schuchter L, Schultz DJ, Synnestvedt M, et al. A prognostic model for predicting 10-year survival in patients with primary melanoma. Ann Intern Med 1996;125:369–375.

CLINICAL PREDICTION RULE

1. Calculate the total points for your patient.

Variable	Points
Constant	−2.245
Lesion thickness (mm)	
<0.76	3.93
0.76–1.69	2.25
1.70–3.60	1.07
Primary lesion on extremity	
Yes	1.47
No	0.0
Age at diagnosis (years)	
≤60	1.1
>60	0.0
Gender	
Male	0.0
Female	0.71
Total:	

The probability of remaining alive at least 10 years = $1/[1 + (1/e^x)]$, where x = the total from above.

2. Another way of looking at the same data.

	10-Year survival			
	Tumor with extremity location		Tumor with nonextremity location	
Variable	Female	Male	Female	Male
Thickness < 0.76 mm				
Age ≤ 60	99%	98%	97%	94%
Age > 60	98%	96%	92%	84%
Thickness 0.76–1.69 mm				
Age ≤ 60	96%	93%	86%	75%
Age > 60	90%	81%	67%	50%
Thickness 1.7–3.6 mm				
Age ≤ 60	89%	80%	65%	48%
Age > 60	73%	57%	38%	24%
Thickness > 3.6 mm				
Age ≤ 60	74%	58%	39%	24%
Age > 60	48%	32%	18%	10%

COAGULOPATHIES

Bleeding Complications of Anticoagulant Therapy

Clinical question

What is the probability of major bleeding in hospitalized patients started on anticoagulant therapy?

Population and setting

Consecutive patients starting long-term anticoagulant treatment in a university hospital were included. Patients were excluded if their partial thromboplastin time (PTT) did not increase by 50% or their prothrombin time (PT) by 2 seconds. The mean age was 62 years; 45% were male.

Study size

There were 411 patients in the training group and 207 in the validation group.

Pretest probability

Of these patients, 4.9% experienced major bleeding.

Type of validation

Grade III: The validation group was a separate sample from the same population, although data for both training and validation groups were gathered at the same time.

Comments

The definition of co-morbidities is subject to misinterpretation. Otherwise, this is a relatively well designed and validated clinical rule.

Reference

Landefeld CS, Cook EF, Flatley M, Weisberg M, Goldman L. Identification and preliminary validation of predictors of major bleeding in hospitalized patients starting anticoagulant therapy. Am J Med 1987;82:703–713.

CLINICAL PREDICTION RULE

1. Calculate the patient's risk score.

Risk factor	Points
Known at the start of therapy	
Co-morbid conditions	
1	1
2	2
3–4	3
Intravenous heparin in elderly patients	
60–79 Years	2
≥80 Years	4
Developing during therapy	
Maximal anticoagulant effect	
PTT or PT 2.0–2.9 × control	1
PT or PTT ≥ 3.0 × control	2
Worsening liver dysfunction	
Yes	4
No	0
Total (13 maximum):	

2. Find your patient's risk of bleeding in the table below.

	Patients with major bleeding	
Point score	Training group	Testing group
0	0% (0/104)	0% (0/55)
1	0% (0/122)	2% (1/61)
2	0% (0/65)	3% (1/35)
3	4% (2/45)	6% (1/16)
4	11% (3/28)	6% (1/17)
5	24% (6/25)	18% (2/11)
6+	36% (8/22)	27% (3/11)

10

Infectious Disease

UPPER RESPIRATORY INFECTIONS

Diagnosis of Streptococcal Pharyngitis (Dobbs' Bayesian Score)

Clinical question

What is the likelihood of streptococcal pharyngitis among patients with sore throat?

Population and setting

Patients over age 4 years with a chief complaint of sore throat presenting to a rural general practice in Ireland were included. Many (42%) were under age 11 years.

Study size

Altogether, 206 patients were studied.

Pretest probability

Of these patients, 35% had streptococcal pharyngitis, a somewhat high percentage (the average prevalence of streptococcal infection among adults with sore throat is only 12%).

Type of validation

Grade IV: The training group was used as the validation group.

Comment

The major problem with this rule, other than its complexity, is the fact that it is based on the observations of a single physician. Although undoubtedly useful and appropriate for Dr. Dobbs, one has to wonder about its generalizability to other practitioners. Also, some of the predictor variables have the potential for ambiguity, including "sore to swallow," "bad smell," and "nose moist." Centor's rule is probably a better choice for the diagnosis of "strep throat."

Reference

Dobbs F. A scoring system for predicting group A streptococcal throat infection. Br J Gen Pract 1996;46:461–464.

CLINICAL PREDICTION RULE

1. Calculate the patient's score, taking the number of points from the appropriate column, depending on whether a symptom or sign is present or absent. For example, if the month is November, add 1 point; if the age is more than 11 years, subtract 1 point; if there is a bad smell, add 2 points; and so on.

Variable	Points if present	Points if absent	Points for your patient
October–December	1	−1	
Age <11 years	2	−1	
Duration <3 days	1	−2	
Very sore throat	1	−2	
Sore to swallow	1	−3	
Bad smell	2	−1	
Ears sore	−3	0	
Cough	−5	1	
Fever	1	−2	
Muscle aches	1	−1	
Flushed	1	−1	
Glands	1	−2	
Exudate	1	−1	
Mouth red/ulcerated	1	−1	
Constant for 35% probability			−2
		Total:	

2. A score higher than −3 had a 71% sensitivity and 71% specificity for prediction of streptococcal pharyngitis.

Strep Score (Centor)

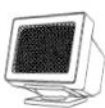

Clinical question

Which patients with a sore throat have streptococcal pharyngitis?

Population and setting

Patients presenting to a university health service with a chief complaint of sore throat were included.

Study size

The validation group had 310 patients.

Pretest probability

Only 5% had streptococcal pharyngitis, slightly lower than average for an adult population (12% is more typical).

Type of validation

Grade I: The validation group was from a distinct population. The rule was developed in one group of patients and validated in another.

Comments

This is a well validated clinical rule and easy to apply in practice. Patients with a high pretest probability can probably be treated empirically, and those with a low probability can be reassured without further testing.

Reference

Poses RM, Cebul RD, Collins M, Fager SS. The importance of disease prevalence in transporting clinical prediction rules. Ann Intern Med 1986;105:586–589.

CLINICAL PREDICTION RULE

1. Count the number of the following clinical characteristics which are present. Give 1 point for each:

History of fever
Anterior cervical adenopathy
Tonsilar exudate
Absence of cough

2. Find the column that most closely matches the pretest likelihood of streptococcal pharyngitis in this patient. The numbers in boldface represent the typical pretest likelihood for adults (12%) and children (33%):

		Pretest probability of streptococcal pharyngitis								
No. of points	Likelihood ratio	5%	10%	**12%**	15%	20%	25%	**33%**	40%	50%
0	0.16	1%	2%	**2%**	2%	3%	5%	**7%**	10%	14%
1	0.30	2%	3%	**4%**	5%	7%	9%	**13%**	17%	23%
2	0.75	4%	8%	**9%**	12%	16%	20%	**27%**	33%	43%
3	2.10	10%	19%	**22%**	27%	34%	41%	**51%**	58%	68%
4	6.30	25%	41%	**46%**	53%	61%	68%	**76%**	81%	86%

Example: a child with history of fever anterior cervical adenopathy, no exudate and cough would have 2 points. His probability of having streptococcal pharyngitis would be found in the row corresponding to 2 points, and the column corresponding to 33%. Hence his probability is 27%.

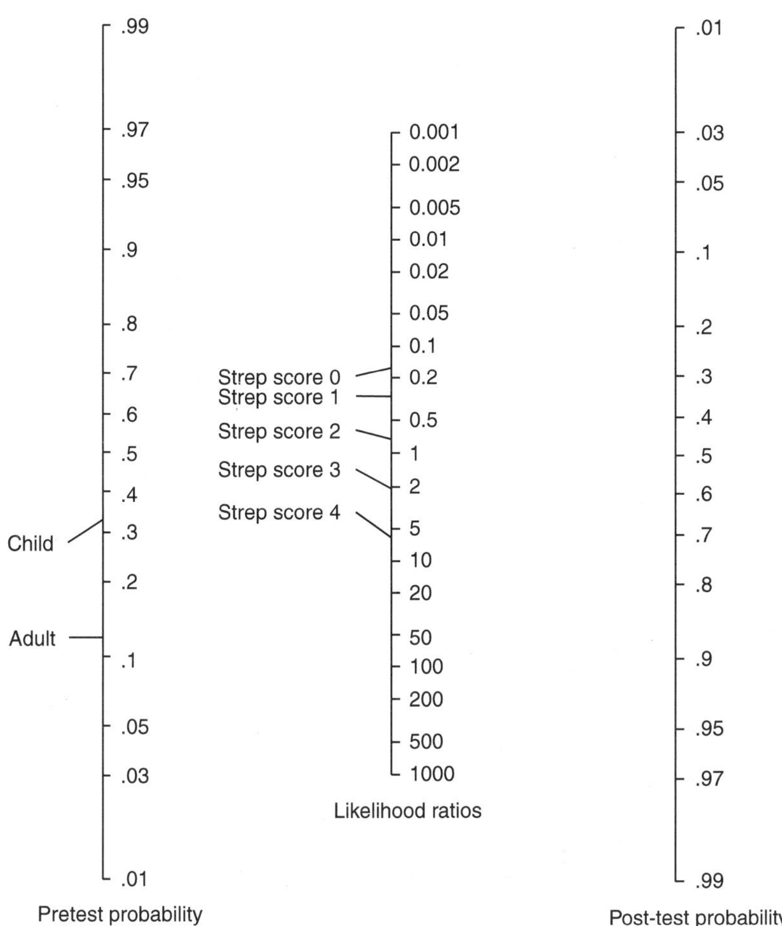
.99
.97
.95
.9
.8
.7
.6
.5
.4
.3
.2
.1
.05
.03
.01
Child
Adult
Pretest probability
0.001
0.002
0.005
0.01
0.02
0.05
0.1
0.2
0.5
1
2
5
10
20
50
100
200
500
1000
Strep score 0
Strep score 1
Strep score 2
Strep score 3
Strep score 4
Likelihood ratios
.01
.03
.05
.1
.2
.3
.4
.5
.6
.7
.8
.9
.95
.97
.99
Post-test probability

Sinusitis Score

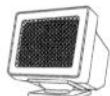

Clinical question

What is the likelihood of acute sinusitis among adult patients with suspected sinusitis?

Population and setting

Adults presenting with suspected sinusitis were included. All patients underwent radiography, and the radiographers were blinded to the clinical findings. The setting was a walk-in clinic of a Veteran's Affairs Medical Center; all patients were men.

Study size

Altogether, 247 patients were studied.

Pretest probability

Of these patients, 38% had sinusitis seen by radiography.

Type of validation

Grade IV: The training group was used as the validation group.

Comment

These are the best data on the diagnosis of acute sinusitis in adults. Unfortunately, the rule has not yet been prospectively validated, so it should be used with caution. The other limitations are that the authors studied only men, and that no children were studied. Interestingly, the clinician's overall impression did quite well, considering that all of these patients had suspected sinusitis.

Reference

Williams JW, Simel DL, Roberts L, Samsa GP. Clinical evaluation for sinusitis: making the diagnosis by history and physical examination. Ann Intern Med 1992;117:705–710.

CLINICAL PREDICTION RULE

1. Count the number of points for your patient to calculate their sinus score.

Clinical finding	Points
Maxillary toothache	1
History of colored nasal discharge	1
No improvement with decongestants	1
Abnormal transillumination using the Mini-Mag Lite flashlight	1
Purulent secretion on examination	1
Total:	

2. The probability of sinusitis is shown below (given an overall probability of 38%).

Sinus score	Likelihood ratio	Probability of sinusitis
0	0.2	9% (5–17%)
1	0.4	21% (15–28%)
2	1.1	40% (33–47%)
3	2.8	63% (53–72%)
4	7.0	81% (69–89%)
5	18.8	92% (81–96%)

Numbers in parentheses are the 95% confidence interval.

3. The clinician's overall impression was also studied (given an overall probability of 38%).

Clinician's overall impression	Likelihood ratio	Probability of sinusitis
High	4.7	72%
Intermediate	1.4	46%
Low	0.4	19%

ENDOCARDITIS

Mortality in Infective Endocarditis

Clinical question

What is the likelihood of death among patients with infective endocarditis?

Population setting

Consecutive patients with infectious endocarditis at a Hong Kong teaching hospital were included. About half were studied retrospectively and half prospectively. Most (n = 120) had rheumatic disease, and 38 had congenital heart disease. Diagnosis was confirmed by blood culture in 170, classic clinical features of infectious endocarditis in 18, and autopsy in 6. Patients undergoing emergency surgery for complicated endocarditis were excluded, as were patients with classic clinical features but negative blood cultures. Only in-hospital mortality was considered. The most common organisms were streptococci (78%) and staphylococci (10%).

Study size

Altogether, 176 patients were studied.

Pretest probability

The mortality rate was 19.9%.

Type of validation

Grade IV: The training group was used as the validation group.

Comments

This rule requires prospective validation before application to patient care.

Reference

Woo KS, Lam YM, Kwok HT, Tse LK, Vallance-Owen J. Prognostic index in prediction of mortality of infective endocarditis. Int J Cardiol 1989;24:47–54.

CLINICAL PREDICTION RULE

1. Determine the number of points for your patient.

Risk factor	Points
Leukocytosis (>10,000 cells/mm^3)	0.5
Congestive heart failure (clinical or radiologic features of pulmonary venous hypertension)	2
Major embolism (cerebral, coronary, splenic, pulmonary, or peripheral)	1.1
Infection with staphylococci, β-hemolytic streptococci, *Pseudomonas* or *Klebsiella*	1.5
Total:	

2. Find your patient's risk of in-hospital death below.

Score	No. of patients	In-hospital mortality
<1.0	104	5.8%
1.0–1.9	19	15.8%
2.0–2.9	30	37.9%
3.0–3.9	9	55.6%
≥4.0	6	83.3%

SEPSIS AND BACTEREMIA

Blood Culture Interpretation

Clinical question

Which blood cultures represent a true positive (i.e., bacteremia)?

Population and setting

Consecutive adult patients who had a positive blood culture at a university hospital were included. The mean age was 51 years; 47% were male.

Study size

The training group had 219 positive blood cultures and the validation group 129.

Pretest probability

Of the positive blood cultures, 44% represented bacteremia. Bacteremia was determined by blinded case review of three infectious disease specialists. They had excellent interrater agreement in their judgments.

Type of validation

Grade II: The validation group was a separate sample from the same population, with data for the validation group gathered prospectively.

Comments

The major limitation of this rule is that some of the predictor variables for the risk score can be misinterpreted: "rapidly fatal disease," "ultimately fatal disease," "acute abdomen."

Reference

Bates DW, Lee TH. Rapid classification of positive blood cultures: prospective validation of a multivariate algorithm. JAMA 1992;267:1962–1966.

CLINICAL PREDICTION RULE

1. Determine your patient's clinical risk score.

Variable	Points
Maximum temperature >38.3°C	3
Rapidly fatal disease (<1 month)	4
Ultimately fatal disease (>1 month but <5 years)	2
Presence of shaking chills	3
Intravenous drug abuse	4
Examination showing acute abdomen	3
Major co-morbidity[a]	3
Total:	

[a]Defined as the presence of any of the following: coma or brain death, bowel perforation, multiple trauma or burns, cardiopulmonary resuscitation within the previous 24 hours, cardiac or bone marrow transplant, severe pancreatitis, acute respiratory distress syndrome, or acute or chronic hepatic failure.

2. Find the risk category based on the number of points.

Points	Risk category
0–2	I
3	II
4–5	III
≥6	IV

3. Add up the number of points for your patient.

Variable	Points
Time until blood culture became positive (days)	
4	2
3	4
2	6
1	8
More than one positive culture	
Yes	7
No	0
Risk category	
I	1
II	2
III	3
IV	4
Organism category	
2 (gram$^+$ cocci in clusters, gram$^+$ rods, mixed, gram$^+$ coccobacilli, or gram-variable rods)	3
3 (gram$^+$ cocci, unclear, or no organisms seen)	7
4 (gram$^+$ cocci in chains)	9
5 (gram$^-$ rods, coagulase$^+$ staphylococci, suspected *Haemophilus,* yeast, fungi, suspected *Neisseria*)	15
Total:	

Gram$^+$, gram$^-$ = gram-positive, gram-negative.

4. Find the likelihood that the culture represents true bacteremia.

Score	No. in group	Bacteremia
0–7	59	14%
8–11	16	19%
12–14	10	70%
>15	44	89%

Probability of Positive Blood Culture in Sepsis Syndrome

Clinical question

Which patients with sepsis syndrome have bacteremia, including prediction of subtypes such as gram-negative, gram-positive, and fungal bloodstream infections?

Population and setting

This was a multicenter study at eight academic tertiary care hospitals. A random sample of adult patients with sepsis syndrome were enrolled using a modification of the standard definition of sepsis (Bone criteria). The average age was 59 years; 58% were male; 61% were on the hospital's medical service; and 21% were of a nonwhite race. The average length of stay was 22 days, with a 66% mean predicted probability of survival using the APACHE III score, so this was a sick group of patients.

Study size

The training group had 881 patients and the validation group 461.

Pretest probability

In the validation group, 31% had bacteremia (13.6% any gram-positive cocci, 10% only gram-positive cocci, 13.5% any gram-negative rods, 11.5% only gram-negative rods, 3.4% any fungi, and 2.5% only fungi).

Type of validation

Grade II: The validation group was a separate sample from the same population, with data for the validation group gathered prospectively.

Comments

This study developed and validated four clinical rules for the prediction of bacteremia. The rule for gram-positive bacteremia was least accurate, and that for gram-negative bacteremia was most useful. The latter rule may be especially helpful when trying to identify patients who might benefit from novel approaches to the treatment of gram-negative sepsis.

Reference

Bates DW, Sands K, Miller E, et al. Predicting bacteremia in patients with sepsis syndrome. J Infect Dis 1997;176:1538–1551.

CLINICAL PREDICTION RULE

Any bacteremia

1. Calculate your patient's risk score.

Risk factor	Points
Suspected or documented focal infection at onset	3
No antibiotics before onset	3
Any liver disease[a]	2
Hickman catheter present	2
Altered mental status within 24 hours	2
Focal abdominal signs within 24 hours	2
Total:	

[a]Cirrhosis with or without portal hypertension, chronic hepatitis within the last 6 months, or hepatic failure with coma or encephalopathy within the last 6 months.

2. Their risk of any bacteremia is shown below for each risk score.

	Risk score (points)				
Parameter	0	1–2	3–4	5–6	≥7
No. with bacteremia	19	11	52	45	26
No. without bacteremia	84	46	106	58	14
Bacteremia[a]	15.0%	18.6%	32.0%	39.6%	64.4%
Likelihood ratio for bacteremia	0.4 (0.3–0.6)[b]	0.5 (0.4–0.7)	0.9 (0.7–1.0)	1.7 (1.4–2.0)	4.4 (3.1–6.2)

[a]Percentages are weighted based on the sampling strategy.
[b]95% Confidence interval.

Any* Staphylococcus aureus *bacteremia

1. Calculate your patient's risk score.

Risk factor	Points
Suspected or documented focal infection with *S. aureus* at onset	2
Hemodialysis before onset	1
Ventilator use before onset	1
Total:	

2. Their risk of any bacteremia is shown below for each risk score.

	Results, by risk score (points)			
Parameter	0	1	2	≥3
No. with bacteremia	9	4	11	5
No. without bacteremia	295	85	42	10
With bacteremia[a]	2.7%	4.6%	19.0%	33.3%
Likelihood ratio for bacteremia	0.5 (0.4–0.7)[b]	0.8 (0.5–1.3)	3.6 (2.6–4.9)	4.9 (2.5–9.0)

[a]Percentages are weighted based on the sampling strategy.
[b]95% Confidence interval.

Any gram-negative rods

1. Calculate your patient's risk score

Risk factor	Points
Total parenteral nutrition before onset	3
No antibiotics before onset	2
History of gram-negative bacteremia	2
Hickman catheter present	1
Focal abdominal signs within 24 hours	1
Chills	1
Total:	

2. Their risk of any bacteremia is shown below for each risk score.

	Results, by risk score (points)				
Parameter	0	1	2	3	≥4
No. with bacteremia	16	13	17	12	5
No. without bacteremia	224	59	71	31	13
Bacteremia[a]	5.7%	20%	17.7%	32.5%	24.8%
Likelihood ratio for bacteremia	0.5 (0.4–0.6)[b]	0.9 (0.6–1.3)	1.3 (1.0–1.7)	2.5 (1.7–3.6)	5.9 (3.6–9.6)

[a]Percentages are weighted based on the sampling strategy.
[b]95% Confidence interval.

Any fungus

1. Calculate your patient's risk score.

Risk factor	Points
Fungal infection at any site	5
Bowel perforation	3
Pyuria	2
Any liver disease[a]	2
Hickman catheter present	2
Altered mental status within 24 hours	2
Total:	

[a]Cirrhosis with or without portal hypertension, chronic hepatitis within the last 6 months, or hepatic failure with coma or encephalopathy within the last 6 months.

2. Their risk of any bacteremia is shown below for each risk score.

	Results, by risk score (points)			
Parameter	0	1–3	4–6	≥7
No. with bacteremia	5	1	5	8
No. without bacteremia	213	160	58	11
Bacteremia[a]	1.9%	0.6%	5.9%	35.9%
Likelihood ratio for bacteremia	0.4 (0.2–0.7)[b]	0.4 0.2–0.7	2.1 (1.2–3.4)	16.5 (10.1–25.9)

[a]Percentages are weighted based on the sampling strategy.
[b]95% Confidence interval.

Probability of Multiresistant Strain in Gram-Negative Bacteremia

Clinical question

Which patients with gram-negative bacteremia are likely to have a multiresistant strain?

Population and setting

All patients over age 13 years at an Israeli medical center who had one or more blood cultures positive for gram-negative bacteremia were included. The age range was 13–99 years.

Study size

There were 286 in the training group and 144 in the validation group.

Pretest probability

Altogether, 21% had a multiresistant strain of bacteria.

Type of validation

Grade II: The validation group was a separate sample from the same population, with data for the validation group gathered prospectively.

Comments

Use of this clinical rule can help tailor empiric antibiotic therapy for patients with a blood culture positive for gram-negative bacteria.

Reference

Leibovici L, Konisberger H, Pitlik SD, Samra Z, Drucker M. Predictive index for optimizing empiric treatment of gram-negative bacteremia. J Infect Dis 1991; 163:193–196.

CLINICAL PREDICTION RULE

1. Count the number of points for your patient.

Variable	Points
Hospital-acquired bacteremia	1
Antibiotic treatment during the month before the bacteremic episode	1
Endotracheal intubation during the month preceding the bacteremic episode	1
Thermal trauma as the cause of hospitalization	1
Total:	

2. Identify their risk for having a multiresistant strain.

No. of points	Multiresistant strains	Pseudomonas strains
0	8%	11%
1	25%	12%
2	64%	28%
3–4	67%	67%

Occult Bacterial Infection in Adults with Unexplained Fever

Clinical question

Which adults with unexplained fever have an occult bacterial infection?

Population and setting

Adults hospitalized in an Israeli department of internal medicine with no clear source of infection after basic investigation during the first day of hospitalization were included. Basic investigation included chest radiograph, detailed history and physical examination, complete blood count, erythrocyte sedimentation rate (ESR), urinalysis, blood chemistry, urine culture, three blood cultures, and other cultures if indicated. If any of the following were found during the first 12 hours of hospitalization, it was regarded as the source of fever, and the patient was excluded: signs of meningeal irritation, erysipelas or cellulitis, exanthem or enanthem, follicular tonsillitis, arthritis, abdominal tenderness and/or other signs of peritoneal irritation, eight or more leukocytes per high-power field on urinalysis, fluid level or opacification of a paranasal sinus, new infiltrate on chest radiograph, positive Gram stain of the phlegm in a patient with respiratory complaints, and signs of symptoms diagnostic of other febrile disease.

Study size

Altogether, 113 patients were studied.

Pretest probability

Of 113 patients, 34 had a bacterial source of fever (15 urinary tract, 3 pneumonia, 2 endocarditis, 2 with bacterial dysentery, 2 with peritoneal infection, 1 ascending cholangitis, 1 bacterial meningitis, 8 bacteremia without obvious source).

Type of validation

Grade I: The validation group was from a distinct population. The rule was developed in one group of patients and validated in another.

Comments

This rule was developed by Mellors and validated by Leibovici et al., a different group of researchers in a different country. It still had good predictive value and may be helpful for identifying patients who can be sent home from the emergency department (group I), those for whom empiric antibiotic therapy may be appropriate (group IV), and those for whom more intensive inpatient investigation is appropriate (groups II and III).

References

Leibovici L, Cohen O, Wysenbeek A. Occult bacterial infection in adults with unexplained fever: validation of a diagnostic index. Arch Intern Med 1990;150:1270–1272.

Mellors JW, Horwitz RI, Harvey MR, Horwitz SM. A simple index to identify occult bacterial infection in adults with acute unexplained fever. Arch Intern Med 1987;147:666–671.

CLINICAL PREDICTION RULE

1. Add up the number of risk factors for your patient.

Risk factor	Points
Age ≥50 years	1
Diabetes mellitus (type I or II)	1
Erythrocyte sedimentation rate ≥30 mm/hr	1
White blood cell count ≥15,000 cells/ml	1
Absolute neutrophil band count ≥1500 cells/ml	1
Total:	

2. Find their risk of occult bacterial infection, bacteremia, and death in the table below.

No. of risk factors	No. of patients in this group	No. with bacterial infection	No. with bacteremia	No. who died
0	11	0	0	0
1	44	12 (27%)	5 (11%)	4 (9%)
2	41	13 (32%)	7 (17%)	4 (10%)
3–5	17	9 (53%)	6 (35%)	5 (29%)
Total:	**113**	**34 (30%)**	**18 (16%)**	**13 (11%)**

MENINGITIS AND CNS INFECTIONS

Probability of Bacterial Meningitis in Adults with Meningitis

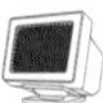

Clinical question

Which adults admitted for suspected meningitis have bacterial infection?

Population and setting

All adult patients admitted with acute meningitis between 1981 and 1990 to one of two Dallas hospitals and three Milwaukee hospitals were included. They were excluded if they were immune-suppressed, had missing data, or the meningitis was associated with a neurosurgical procedure. The mean age was 42 years; 64.3% were male.

Study size

There were 120 in the original study's training group and 160 in the validation group (McKinney). The validation study (Hoen) had 398 patients in the validation group.

Pretest probability

In the training group, 38.3% had bacterial meningitis; the remainder had viral meningitis. In the validation group, 29% had bacterial meningitis.

Type of validation

Grade I: The validation group was from a distinct population. The rule was developed in one group of patients and validated in another.

Comments

This is a well validated rule, but the calculations are complex. To apply it, program it into a calculator, spreadsheet, or handheld computer, or use the included software. The area under the ROC curve for this rule was approximately 0.99, which is outstanding. Note that in the validation study 102 patients were not included because the diagnosis of bacterial versus viral meningitis was not reliable.

Reference

Hoen B, Viel JF, Paquot C, et al. Multivariate approach to differential diagnosis of acute meningitis. Eur J Clin Microbiol Infect Dis 1995;14:267–274.

McKinney WP, Heudebert GR, Harper SA, Young MJ, McIntir DD. Validation of a clinical prediction rule for the differential diagnosis of acute meningitis. J Gen Intern Med 1994;9:8–12.

CLINICAL PREDICTION RULE

1. Calculate the patient's total score.

Variable	Value	Multiplied by	Total
Months from August 1 (maximum 12)		0.52	
CSF/Blood glucose ratio (maximum 0.6)		−12.76	
PMN count in CSF (10^3/mL)[a]		$(0.341) \times (\text{value})^{0.333}$	
Age (years)			
≤1		2.29	
>1 and ≤2		−2.71	
>2 and ≤22		−0.159	
>22		0.100	
Constant (by age in years)			
≤1 year			2.79
>1 and ≤2 years			7.79
>2 and ≤22 years			2.69
>22 years			−3.01
		Total:	

[a]Range 0–29,700 in bacterial meningitis and 0–1260 in viral meningitis.
CSF = cerebrospinal fluid; PMN = polymorphonuclear neutrophils.

Example: A 20-year-old presenting in October with a CSF blood glucose ratio of 0.5 and PMN count of 3000/ml would have the following score:

$$(2 \times 0.52) + (0.5 \times -12.76) + (0.341 \times 3^{0.333}) + (20 \times -0.159) + 2.69$$

2. The probability of acute bacterial meningitis is calculated from the equation below.

$$\text{Probability} = 1/[1 + (1/e^{\text{total}})]$$

A probability >0.5 is 94% sensitive and 97% specific [positive likelihood ratio (LR^+) = 31.3; negative likelihood ratio (LR^-) = 0.06)] for the diagnosis of acute bacterial meningitis in patients with meningitis.

Prognosis for Meningococcal Meningitis

Clinical question

What is the prognosis for patients with meningococcal disease?

Population and setting

In this Spanish study (Barcelona), patients from one of 24 hospitals with a positive blood or cerebrospinal fluid (CSF) culture for *Neisseria meningitidis* were included. In the training group the mean age was 12.4 years (range 31 days to 89 years); 46% were male. In the validation group the mean age was 12.7 years (range 45 days to 81 years); 44% were male. The training group consisted of patients recruited from 1987 through 1990, and the validation group patients recruited in 1991 and 1992.

Study size

The training group had 624 patients and the validation group 283.

Pretest probability

Of patients in the validation group, 6.0% died.

Type of validation

Grade II: The validation group was a separate sample from the same population, with data for the validation group gathered prospectively.

Comments

This is the best validated prognostic model for patients with meningococcal meningitis. It can help guide the use of aggressive therapy, although it should certainly not be the only determinant of the aggressiveness of therapy. Note that this study included only patients with microbiologic proof of disease. Cases where antibiotics are given in the prehospital setting and microbiologic proof is compromised generally have a better prognosis and may not be applicable for this rule.

Reference

Barquet N, Domingo P, Cayla JA, et al. Prognostic factors in meningococcal disease: development of a bedside predictive model and scoring system. JAMA 1997; 278:491–496.

CLINICAL PREDICTION RULE

1. Calculate your patient's risk score (range −1 to 4).

Risk factor	Points
Preadmission antibiotics given	−1
Age (years)	
15–59	0
≥60	1
Focal neurologic signs[a]	1
Hemorrhagic diathesis[b]	2
Total:	

[a]Motor, sensory, or cranial nerve disturbances of central origin that were not present before the episode of meningococcal disease.

[b]Spontaneous clinically apparent bleeding, including bleeding from wounds, hematoma, hematuria, spontaneous gingival bleeding, epistaxis, or gastrointestinal or gynecologic bleeding together with perivenipuncture bruises or venipuncture bleeding. This determination was made irrespective of the presence of petechiae and once prior coagulation disorders or anticoagulant therapy had been ruled out by assessing the patient's medical history.

2. The risk of death is shown in the table below.

Risk score	No. of patients in this group	Mortality
−1	287	0%
0	533	2.3%
1	55	27.3%
≥2	32	75.0%

11

Musculoskeletal System

OSTEOPOROSIS

Risk of Low Bone Density in a Screening Population

Clinical question

Which women are at risk for low bone mineral density (BMD)?

Population and setting

Patients came from 106 sites; 50% of the physicians were generalists. Women were included if over age 45 and postmenopausal (amenorrheic for at least 6 months). They were excluded if they had significant scoliosis, trauma, or sequelae of orthopedic procedures prohibiting BMD measurements, metabolic bone disease other than osteoporosis, metastatic cancer to bone, or renal impairment.

Study size

The training group had 1279 women and the validation set 207.

Pretest probability

Low BMD (2 SD or more below the mean for young, healthy white women) was found in 44% of the validation cohort at the hip, 21% at the spine, and 17% at both hip and spine.

Type of validation

Grade II: The validation group was a separate sample from the same population, with data for the validation group gathered prospectively.

Comments

This simple score can help identify women at high risk for low BMD. It has higher sensitivity than specificity, appropriate for such a screening test. Of course, given the inconvenience, side effects, and cost of pharmacologic treatment, it is important to consider whether the results of screening would change anything for a patient already exercising, taking adequate vitamin D and calcium, and using hormone replacement therapy.

Reference

Lydick E, Cook K, Turpin J, et al. Development and validation of a simple questionnaire to facilitate identification of women likely to have low bone density. Am J Managed Care 1998;4:37–48.

CLINICAL PREDICTION RULE

1. Add up the points for your patient.

Risk factor	Points
Race is *not* Black	5
Rheumatoid arthritis	4
History of wrist fracture(s)	4
History of rib fracture(s)	4
History of hip fracture(s)	4
First digit of age × 3[a]	
Never received estrogen therapy	1
(Weight/10) × −1, truncated to integer[b]	
Total:	

[a]If a woman is 58, enter 5 × 3 = 15. If she is 64, enter 6 × 3 = 18.
[b]For a weight of 126 pounds, enter 12 × −1 = −12. For a weight of 87 pounds, enter 8 × −1 = −8.

Example: A 126-pound, 67-year-old white woman with a history of rheumatoid arthritis, a history of hip fracture, and a history of estrogen therapy would have a score of 19: $5 + 4 + 0 + 0 + 4 + (6 \times 3) + 0 - (12 \times 1) = 19$.

2. A score >6 is 91% sensitive and 40% specific for low BMD. That is, 91% of patients with low BMD have a score >6, and 40% of healthy women will have a score ≤6. The corresponding positive likelihood ratio (LR^+) is 1.5, and the negative likelihood ratio (LR^-) is 0.2. The rule is therefore better at ruling out osteoporosis when negative than it is at ruling in the condition when positive.

ACUTE FRACTURES

Knee Injuries (Ottawa Knee Rule)

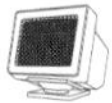

Clinical question

Which knee injuries require a radiographic series for evaluation?

Population and setting

Adult patients presenting with acute knee injury to one of two university hospital emergency departments in Canada were included. The mean age was 37 years (range 18–91 years); 55% were male.

Study size

The validation group had 1096 patients.

Pretest probability

Altogether, 6% had a clinically important fracture.

Type of validation

Grade II: The validation group was a separate sample from the same population, with data for the validation group gathered prospectively.

Comments

This is a well validated clinical rule that can reduce the use of radiography for traumatic knee injuries.

Reference

Stiell IG, Greenberg GH, Wells GA, et al. Prospective validation of a clinical prediction rule for the use of radiography in acute knee injuries. JAMA 1996;275:611–615.

CLINICAL PREDICTION RULE

A radiographic examination is required only for acute knee injury patients with one or more of these findings related to age, tenderness, or function:

Age 55 years or older *or*
Tenderness at the head of the fibula *or*
Isolated tenderness of the patella (no bone tenderness of the knee other than the patella) *or*
Inability to flex to 90 degrees *or*
Inability to bear weight immediately and in the emergency department (four steps), that is, unable to transfer weight twice onto each lower limb regardless of limping

This rule has a sensitivity of 100% (identifies all patients with fracture), 49% specificity, 11% positive predictive value (11% with a positive test actually have a fracture), and 100% negative predictive value. The positive likelihood ratio is 2.0, and the negative likelihood ratio is 0.01.

Ankle Injuries (Ottawa Ankle Rule)

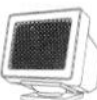

Clinical question

Which ankle injuries require a radiographic series for evaluation?

Population and setting

Consecutive adult patients presenting with ankle injury to one of two university hospital emergency departments were included. The mean age was 36 years (range 18–92 years); 52% were male.

Study size

The training group had 750 patients; 1032 were used to refine the rule and 453 to test it.

Pretest probability

A clinically significant fracture near the malleolus was seen in 11%.

Type of validation

Grade II: The validation group was a separate sample from the same population, with data for the validation group gathered prospectively.

Comments

The Ottawa Ankle Rule is a model for how to both develop and validate a rule. It is widely used in emergency departments, although training is necessary to achieve the accuracy demonstrated by Stiell et al.

Reference

Stiell IG, Greenberg GH, McKnight RD, et al. Clinical prediction rules for the use of radiography in acute ankle injuries: refinement and prospective validation. JAMA 1993;269:1127–1132.

CLINICAL PREDICTION RULE

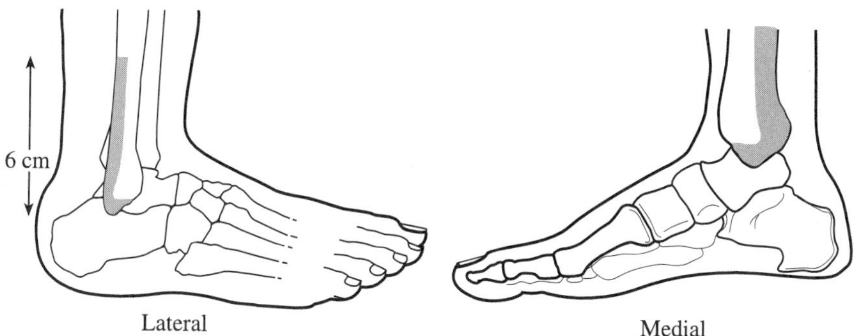

An ankle radiographic series is necessary only if there is pain near the malleoli *and* any of these findings:

1. Inability to bear weight both immediately and in the emergency department (four steps)
2. Bone tenderness at the posterior edge or tip of either malleolus

This rule has a sensitivity of 100% (all patients with fracture identified) and specificity of 79%. The positive likelihood ratio is 4.8, and the negative likelihood ratio is 0.01.

Midfoot Injuries (Ottawa Foot Rule)

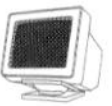

Clinical question

Which foot injuries require a radiographic series for evaluation?

Population and setting

Consecutive adult patients presenting with ankle injury to one of two university emergency departments were included. The mean age was 36 years (range 18–92 years); 52% were male.

Study size

The training group had 750 patients; 1032 were used to refine the rule and 453 to test it.

Pretest probability

A clinically significant fracture in the midfoot was seen in 4%.

Type of validation

Grade II: The validation group was a separate sample from the same population, with data for the validation group gathered prospectively.

Comments

This rule was developed in parallel with the Ottawa Ankle Rules. It is well validated, but its use depends on some training for clinicians to do it accurately.

Reference

Stiell IG, Greenberg GH, McKnight RD, et al. Clinical prediction rules for the use of radiography in acute ankle injuries: refinement and prospective validation. JAMA 1993;269:1127–1132.

CLINICAL PREDICTION RULE

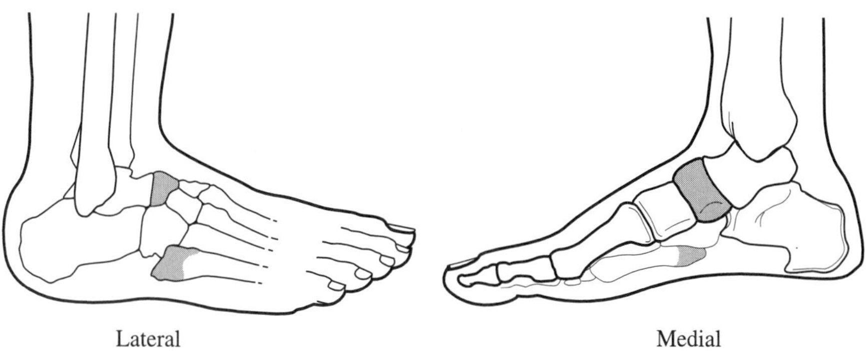

A foot radiographic series is necessary only if there is pain in the midfoot *and* any of these findings:

1. Inability to bear weight both immediately and in the emergency department (four steps)
2. Bone tenderness at the navicular or the base of the fifth metatarsal

This rule has a sensitivity of 100% (all patients with fracture identified) and specificity of 79%. The positive likelihood ratio is 4.8, and the negative likelihood ratio is 0.01.

Knee Injuries (Pittsburgh Knee Rules)

Clinical question

Which patients with acute knee injury require radiography?

Population and setting

A convenience sample of patients presenting with acute knee injuries requiring radiography over an 18-month period were included. Blunt trauma included that incurred by falling to the ground.

Study size

Altogether, 745 patients were studied.

Pretest probability

Of these patients, 91 had a fracture (12.2%).

Type of validation

Grade I: The validation group was from a distinct population. The rule was developed in one group of patients and validated in another. Radiography was ordered according to the usual practice of individual physicians, so some patients with knee injury were not radiographed, and injury may have been missed.

Comments

This rival to the Ottawa Knee Rules is quite accurate. However, the reference standard (radiography) was not applied to all patients, and the patients were a convenience sample rather than a consecutive sample. Both of these issues can inflate the accuracy of the rule.

Reference

Seaberg DC, Yealy DM, Lukens T, Auble T, Mathias S. Multicenter comparison of two clinical decision rules for the use of radiography in acute high-risk injuries. Ann Emerg Med 1998;32:8–13.

CLINICAL PREDICTION RULE

1. Use this algorithm to determine whether a knee radiograph is needed.

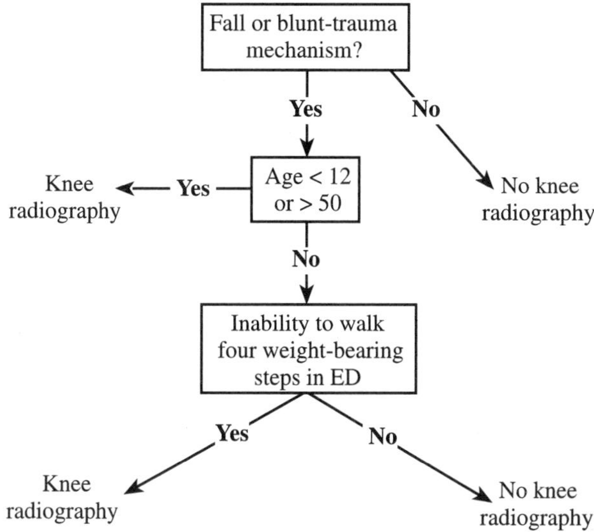

2. The accuracy of the rule is shown below.

Patient group	Fracture	No fracture
Fracture predicted by rule	90	264
Fracture not predicted by rule	1	390

The rule is 99% sensitive (i.e., it detects 99% of fractures, with a 95% confidence interval of 94–100%) and 60% specific. The positive likelihood ratio is 1.7, and the negative likelihood ratio is 0.02.

HIP FRACTURE/FALLING

Risk of Falls in Hospitalized Elderly

Clinical question

Which elderly hospitalized patients are at an especially high risk of falling?

Population and setting

The rule was developed using data from 116 elderly patients who had fallen (mean age 85) and the 116 patients in the bed next to them who had not. It was evaluated in 217 patients at the same hospital (local validation) and 331 in the acute and rehabilitation wards of another British hospital (remote validation).

Study size

The training group had 232 patients and the validation groups 217 (local) and 331 (remote).

Pretest probability

The percentage of patients falling was 33% in the local validation group and 24% in the remote validation group.

Type of validation

Grade I/II: The remote validation group was from a distinct population; that is, the rule was developed in one group of patients and validated in another. The local validation group was a prospective sample from the same hospital where the rule was developed.

Comments

This simple rule helps identify patients at higher than average risk of falling. The remote validation results are more likely to resemble those in your institution. The results shown below include only the remote validation; for the local validation findings see the original article.

Reference

Oliver D, Britton M, Seed P, et al. Development and evaluation of evidence based risk assessment tool (STRATIFY) to predict which elderly inpatients will fall: case-control and cohort studies. BMJ 1997;315:1049–1053.

CLINICAL PREDICTION RULE

1. Add up the number of points for your patient.

Risk factor	Points
Presented with a fall or has fallen since admission	1
Agitation	1
Major visual impairment	1
Frequent urination needs	1
Poor transfer and mobility	1
Total:	

2. Determine the risk of falling.

		Probability of fall	
Score	Likelihood ratio for falling (remote validation)	Given population risk of 20%	Given population risk of 30%
0–1	0.1	2.4%	4.1%
≥2	2.9	42.0%	55.4%
0–2	0.5	11.1%	17.6%
≥3	4.4	52.4%	65.3%

Note that a score of 0–1 means that falling is unlikely, whereas a score of ≥3 puts a patient at significant risk for falling. A score of 2 is less useful clinically.

Risk of Hip Fracture

Clinical question

Which elderly white women are at risk for hip fracture?

Population and setting

Women aged 65 years or older who had no previous hip fracture were recruited through population-based mailings in Portland, Oregon; Minneapolis; Baltimore; and the Monongahela Valley, Pennsylvania. Women who had experienced a previous fracture or who could not walk were excluded.

Study size

Altogether, 9516 women were studied.

Pretest probability

In all, 192 women (2%) had a hip fracture not due to a motor vehicle accident during the 4-year follow-up period

Type of validation

Grade IV: The training group was used as the validation group.

Comments

This clinical rule was developed in a population of white women; black women were excluded because of their low incidence of hip fracture. Although not prospectively validated, the methods were otherwise sound, and it was developed from a representative sample of patients. The major practical limitation is the need to estimate contrast sensitivity and depth perception. References are given for obtaining these instruments.

Reference

Cummings SR, Nevitt MC, Browner WS, et al. Risk factors for hip fracture in white women. N Engl J Med 1995;332:767–773.

CLINICAL PREDICTION RULE

1. Add up the number of the following risk factors your patient has.

Risk factor	Points
Age >80 years	1
Maternal history of hip fracture	1
Any fracture (except hip fracture) since age 50	1
Fair, poor, or very poor health[a]	1
Previous hyperthyroidism	1
Anticonvulsant therapy	1
Current long-acting benzodiazepine therapy	1
Current weight less than at the age of 25	1
Height at the age of 25 ≥ 168 cm (5′ 6″)	1
Caffeine intake more than the equivalent of two cups of coffee per day	1
On feet ≤4 hours a day	1
No walking for exercise	1
Inability to rise from chair without using arms	1
Poor depth perception (lowest quartile)[b]	1
Poor contrast sensitivity (lowest quartile)[c]	1
Total:	

[a]Health was self-rated as very poor, poor, fair, good, or excellent.
[b]Howard-Dolman device (Gibson JJ. In: *The Perception of the Visual World.* Boston: Houghton Mifflin, 1950.)
[c]Ginsburg AP. A new contrast sensitivity vision test chart. Am J Optom Physiol Opt 1984;64:403–407.

2. The risk of hip fracture is as follows.

No. of risk factors	Rate of hip fracture (no./1000 woman-years)
0–2	4.8
3–4	11.5
≥5	51.4

3. If you have the calcaneal bone density, you can make a more precise estimate of risk. Find the number of risk factors in the left hand column and the rate of hip fracture (per 1000 woman-years) in the appropriate column corresponding to the tertile calcaneal bone density.

	Risk of hip fracture (no./1000 woman-years)		
No. of risk factors	Lowest third calcaneal bone density	Middle third calcaneal bone density	Highest third calcaneal bone density
0–2	3.3	3.3	7.8
3–4	5.7	16.8	12.0
≥5	28.2	44.1	81.9

Need for Transfusion after Joint Replacement

Clinical question

What is the likelihood that a patient undergoing knee or hip replacement will require a blood transfusion?

Population and setting

This rule was validated in two Canadian hospitals. The mean age at both hospitals was approximately 48 years; 48% were male at the first and 38% at the second. Approximately 55% of patients had total knee arthroplasty and 45% total hip replacement.

Study size

The validation group had 460 patients.

Pretest probability

The probability of transfusion was 37.0% at site 2 and 7.4% at site 1.

Type of validation

Grade I: The test set was from a distinct population. The rule was developed in one group of patients and validated in another.

Comments

Despite the differences in the populations at the two hospitals and the large difference in baseline transfusion rates, the clinical rule performed well at both sites.

Reference

Larocque BJ, Gilbert K, Brien WF. Prospective validation of a point score system for predicting blood transfusion following hip or knee replacement. Transfusion 1998;38: 932–937.

CLINICAL PREDICTION RULE

1. Calculate the risk score.

Risk factor	Points
Hemoglobin (g/L)	
>130	0
111–130	2
≤110	3
Weight (kg)	
>100	0
81–100	1
≤80	2
Surgery	
Knee	0
Hip	2
Bilateral knee	3
Bilateral hip	6
Primary or revision	
Primary	0
Revision	2
Total:	

2. Find the risk of transfusion.

	Site 1 (overall rate 7.4%)		Site 2 (overall rate 36.8%)	
Risk score	No. of patients	% Transfused	No. of patients	% Transfused
≤2	92	3.3% (0–7)	99	14% (7–21)
3–4	89	2.2% (0–5)	73	44% (32–55)
5–7	45	22% (10–34)	50	60% (46–74)
≥8	3	67% (13–100)	9	100% (NA)

Prolonged Nursing Home Stay after Hip Fracture

Clinical question

What is the probability that a patient with hip fracture will have a prolonged nursing home stay?

Population and setting

The training population consisted of patients with hip fracture between 1991 and 1994, at a stratified random sample of 27 rehabilitation facilities and 65 nursing homes from 17 states. All patients were over age 65 and were Medicare beneficiaries. The validation group consisted of patients admitted to five integrated fee-for-service health systems or six health maintenance organizations (HMOs) with "Medicare risk" contracts between 1993 and 1995. The mean age of both groups was approximately 81 years; approximately 85% were female.

Study size

The training group had 364 patients and the validation group 279.

Pretest probability

The overall probability of nursing home residence at 6 months was 6.1% in the validation group and 18.7% in the training group.

Type of validation

Grade I: The test set was from a distinct population. The rule was developed in one group of patients and validated in another.

Comments

It is striking how different the pretest probability was between the training and validation groups. Because the area under the ROC curve was similarly good between the training and validation groups (0.84 vs. 0.81), results for both groups are presented.

Reference

Steiner JF, Kramer AM, Eilertsen TB, Kowalsky JC. Development and validation of a clinical prediction rule for prolonged nursing home residence after hip fracture. J Am Geriatr Soc 1997;45:1510–1514.

CLINICAL PREDICTION RULE

1. Calculate your patient's risk score.

Patient characteristic	Points
Unmarried	1
Bowel or bladder incontinence	1
Dependence for ambulation	1
Cognitive impairment (Mini-Mental State score < 24)	1
Total:	

2. Find their risk of still being in the nursing home 6 months after admission for rehabilitation.

	Training group		Validation group	
Risk score	No.	In nursing home at 6 months	No.	In nursing home at 6 months
4	41	73.2%	8	50.0%
3	56	30.4%	39	15.4%
2	115	11.3%	77	2.6%
1	107	3.7%	85	2.4%
0	25	0%	30	0%

■ HEAD, NECK, AND SPINE INJURIES

CT for Head Injury

Clinical question

Which head-injured patients due to acute trauma require cranial computed tomography (CT)?

Population and setting

All patients with acute head trauma presenting to an urban emergency department who underwent head CT during the study period were included: 46% were age 13–30 years, 34% were 31–59 years, and 20% were 60 years or older; 68% were male.

Study size

There were 540 patients in the training group and 273 in the validation group.

Pretest probability

Of the patients in the validation group, 16% had a clinically significant lesion.

Type of validation

Grade II: The validation group was a separate sample from the same population, with data for the validation group gathered prospectively.

Comments

This rule helps identify head-injury patients who are at low risk for clinically important abnormalities on head CT. It is not perfect, though, and should be used with that in mind and in concern with other clinical information. Absence of any of these risk factors does not completely rule out abnormal CT.

Reference

Madden C, Witzke DB, Sanders AB, Valente J, Fritz M. High-yield selection criteria for cranial computed tomography after acute trauma. Acad Emerg Med 1995;2:248–253.

CLINICAL PREDICTION RULE

1. Patients with *none* of the following criteria are at low risk for an abnormal head CT:

History of loss of consciousness (LOC)
LOC >5 minutes
Inappropriate level of consciousness
Combativeness
Decreasing level of consciousness
Facial injury
Penetrating skull injury
Palpable depressed skull fracture
Acute pupillary inequality
Signs of basilar skull fracture
Glasgow Coma Scale score <15

2. Applying these criteria identifies a low risk group. The rule has 96% sensitivity, 21% specificity, 19% positive predictive value, and 96% negative predictive value for detecting clinically significant findings on CT. That is, 96% of patients with an abnormal head CT have at least one of the above abnormalities. Also, 19% of patients with one of these abnormalities will have an abnormal CT, and 96% with none of these abnormalities will have a normal head CT.

Identifying Low Risk for Cervical Spine Injury

Clinical question

Which patients with a chief complaint of blunt trauma are at low risk for cervical spine fracture?

Population and setting

Consecutive blunt trauma patients presenting to the emergency department for whom a cervical spine radiograph was ordered were included. The median age was 25 years (range 6 months to 98 years); 59% were male.

Study size

There were 974 patients in the validation group.

Pretest probability

Altogether, 2.8% had a cervical spine fracture (27 of 974).

Type of validation

Grade I: The validation group was from a distinct population. The rule was developed empirically from the literature and validated in another.

Comments

This rule was well validated in an emergency department setting. It is easy to apply and can help identify patients at low risk of cervical spine injury. Of course no rule is perfect, and even patients predicted to be at low risk could have a cervical spine injury.

Reference

Hoffman JR, Schriger DL, Mower W, Luo JS, Zucker M. Low-risk criteria for cervical-spine radiography in blunt trauma: a prospective study. Ann Emerg Med 1992;21: 1454–1460.

CLINICAL PREDICTION RULE

1. Does your patient have any of the following risk factors for cervical spine injury?

Midline neck tenderness
Altered level of alertness
Another severely painful injury
Evidence of intoxication

2. Interpretation: Patients with any of the above require cervical spine radiography. This criterion had 100% sensitivity for the detection of cervical spine fracture. Patients without any of these risk factors had a 100% negative predictive value for cervical spine fracture (i.e., none had a fracture) in the validation study.

Risk for Disability and Functional Limitation from Back Pain

Clinical question

Which patients with back pain are at high risk for long-term functional limitations and disability?

Population and setting

Adult patients presenting to a primary care physician at Group Health Cooperative in Puget Sound were eligible, and 72% agreed to participate. Patients were followed for 2 years, and 92% completed the study.

Study size

The training group had 569 patients and the validation group 644.

Pretest probability

Of the patients in the validation group, 15% had long-term functional disability.

Type of validation

Grade II: The validation group was a separate sample from the same population, with data for the validation group gathered prospectively.

Comments

Although somewhat complicated, this rule could be built into the evaluation of patients with back pain to identify those at high risk for major functional limitation. They could then undergo more aggressive counseling and physical therapy.

Reference

Dionne CE, Koepsell TD, Korff MV, et al. Predicting long-term functional limitations among back pain patients in primary care settings. J Clin Epidemiol 1997;50:31–41.

CLINICAL PREDICTION RULE

1. Add the socres for each depression screening question below. Do not include questions answered "don't know".

Question	Not at all	A little bit	Moderately	Quite a bit	Extremely	Don't know
In the past month, how much were you distressed by:						
Worrying too much about things	0	1	2	3	4	0
Feeling no interest in things	0	1	2	3	4	0
Feelings of worthlessness	0	1	2	3	4	0
Feelings of guilt	0	1	2	3	4	0
Feeling lonely or blue	0	1	2	3	4	0
Feeling low in energy or slowed down	0	1	2	3	4	0
Sleep that is restless or disturbed	0	1	2	3	4	0
Feeling everything is an effort	0	1	2	3	4	0
Blaming yourself for things	0	1	2	3	4	0
Feeling hopeless about the future	0	1	2	3	4	0
	Total:					

2. Divide the score above by the number of questions answered (do not include questions answered "don't know"). This is the *depression score.*

3. Add the scores for each somatization screening question below. Do not include questions answered "don't know."

Question	Not at all	A little bit	Moderately	Quite a bit	Extremely	Don't know
In the past month, how much were you distressed by:						
Faintness or dizziness	0	1	2	3	4	0
A lump in your throat	0	1	2	3	4	0
Feeling weak in parts of your body	0	1	2	3	4	0
Heavy feelings in your arms or legs	0	1	2	3	4	0
Trouble getting your breath	0	1	2	3	4	0
Hot or cold spells	0	1	2	3	4	0
Numbness or tingling in parts of your body	0	1	2	3	4	0
	Total:					

4. Divide the score above by the number of questions answered (do not include questions answered "don't know"). This is the *somatization score.*

5. Find the combination of *depression score* and *somatization score* in the table below to determine the risk of major long-term functional limitation.

Depression score	Somatization score	No. of patients in this group	With major functional limitation
<0.444	Any	147	2.0%
0.444–1.5	<0.333	85	1.2%
0.444–1.5	≥0.333	154	19.5%
>1.5	Any	85	42.4%

Prediction of Outcome after Lumbar Spine Surgery

Clinical question

Which patients undergoing lumbar spine surgery for disc disease will have a good outcome 2 years later?

Population and setting

Two university hospitals, one in Germany and one in Switzerland, were the setting. All patients were under age 70 and spoke German. The mean age was approximately 45 years; 55% of the patients were male; and only about one-fourth had undergone previous spine surgery. In all, 51% of patients had disc disease only, 18% had disc disease plus another diagnosis such as osteoarthritis or spinal stenosis, and 31% had surgery for reasons other than disc disease. Patient selection was nonconsecutive.

Study size

The prediction rule was developed in a group of 381 patients in a previous study and validated in a group of 164, of whom 134 were followed for 2 years.

Pretest probability

Of the 134 patients, 56 had a good outcome at 2 years. Of the 88 patients with disc disease, 43 had a good outcome.

Type of validation

Grade I: The validation group was from a distinct population. The rule was developed in one group of patients and validated in another.

Comments

Outcomes were different for the three groups of patients, so it is important to consider your patient's indications for surgery. In particular, the score was not helpful in patients without disc disease. An important limitation of this rule is the lack of clear definition of terms such as "job level," "pain in other locations," and "deficiency of reflexes." It is therefore most useful as a research tool and is of limited use in clinical practice.

Reference

Junge A, Frohlich M, Ahrens S, et al. Predictors of bad and good outcome of lumbar spine surgery. Spine 1996;21:1056–1065.

CLINICAL PREDICTION RULE

1. Calculate your patient's score.

Variable	Points
Duration of reduced working ability (weeks)	
≤2	−3
>2 to 26	0
>26 to 52	1
>52	3
Duration of acute back pain (weeks)	
≤2	−2
>2 to 12	0
>12 to 26	1
>26	3
Number of other pain locations	
0	−1
1	1
2	3
>2	6
Disability pension considered or applied	
No	0
Yes	3
Depression (Beck Depression Inventory)	
≤10 points	0
>10 points	1
Intensity of pain using a visual analogue scale (VAS) (0 = no pain, 10 = unbearable pain)	
<2	−4
≥2	0
Job level	
Low	1
Middle	0
High	−2
Deficiency of reflexes	
No	1
Yes	0
Additional diagnosis	
No	0
Yes	1
Total:	

2. Find the score in the left-hand column and the number of patients with each type of outcome in the next three columns.

	No. with this outcome		
Score	Good	Moderate	Bad
<0	19	7	0
0–1	10	1	3
2–5	11	5	9
6–10	3	4	9
>10	0	0	4

Good outcome = none of these criteria; moderate outcome = one of the criteria, or two of the criteria, if back pain is little (VAS 0–3); bad outcome = all three criteria or two criteria and moderate back pain (VAS ≥ 4).

Three criteria were used to define the outcome: severe low back pain (VAS ≥ 6), reduced working ability of more than half a year or no return to previous job, and frequent visits to the physician or hospital stay.

■ LIMB SALVAGE

Limb Salvage Surgery

Clinical question

Which patients with major lower extremity trauma and vascular injury are likely to benefit from limb salvage surgery?

Population and setting

Consecutive patients having sustained major lower extremity arterial damage presenting to a university medical center between 1985 and 1990. The mean age was 32 years (range 9–76 years) 75% were male.

Study size

Altogether, 70 limbs in 67 patients were studied.

Pretest probability

In all, 27% of limbs were eventually amputated.

Type of validation

Grade IV: The training group was used as the validation group. The index was empirically developed, though, and did not appear to rely much on the training group.

Comments

This small study provides some guidance in the determination of prognosis for limb salvage surgery. However, it was not prospectively validated and should only be used with caution.

Reference

Russell WL, Sailors DM, Whittle TB, Fisher DF, Burns RP. Limb salvage versus traumatic amputation: a decision based on a seven part predictive index. Ann Surg 1991;213:473–481.

CLINICAL PREDICTION RULE

1. Add up the points for your patient.

Location	Extent of injury	Points
Artery	Contusion, intimal tear, partial laceration or avulsion (pseudoaneurysm) with no distal thrombosis and palpable pedal pulses; complete occlusion of three shank vessels or profunda	0
	Occlusion of two or more shank vessels, complete laceration, avulsion or thrombosis of femoral or popliteal vessels without palpable pedal pulses	1
	Complete occlusion of femoral, popliteal, or three of three shank vessels with no distal runoff available	2
Nerve	Contusion or stretch injury; minimal clean laceration of femoral, peroneal, or tibial nerve	0
	Partial transection or avulsion of sciatic nerve; complete or partial transection of femoral, peroneal, or tibial nerve	1
	Complete transection or avulsion of sciatic nerve; complete transection or avulsion of both peroneal and tibial nerves	2
Bone	Closed fracture one or two sites; open fracture without comminution or with minimal displacement; closed dislocation without fracture; open joint without foreign body; fibula fracture	0
	Closed fracture at three or more sites on same extremity; open fracture with comminution or moderate to large displacement; segmental fracture; fracture dislocation; open joint with foreign body; bone loss < 3 cm	1
	Bone loss > 3 cm; type IIIB or IIIC fracture (open fracture with periosteal stripping, gross contamination, extensive soft tissue injury or loss)	2
Skin	Clean laceration single or multiple, or small avulsion injuries, all with primary repair; first degree burn	0
	Delayed closure due to contamination; large avulsion requiring split-thickness skin graft or flap closure; second and third degree burns.	1
Muscle	Laceration or avulsion involving a single compartment or single tendon	0
	Laceration or avulsion involving two or more compartments; complete laceration or avulsion of two or more tendons	1
	Crush injury	2
Deep vein	Contusion, partial laceration, or avulsion; complete laceration or avulsion if alternate route of venous return is intact; superficial vein injury	0
	Complete laceration, avulsion, or thrombosis with no alternate route of venous return	1
Warm ischemia time	<6 hours	0
	6–9 hours	1
	9–12 hours	2
	12–15 hours	3
	>15 hours	4
	Total:	

2. The outcome for 70 injured limbs is shown below.

Limb salvage index	Limb salvage	Secondary/functional amputation	Primary amputation
0	7		
1	13		
2	14		
3	8		
4	5		
5	4		
6		4	
7		2	3
8		1	5
9		1	3

12

Neurology/Psychiatry

DEMENTIA

Prediction of Activities of Daily Living Dependence in Elderly Adults

Clinical question

Which independent-living older adults will develop dependence for their activities of daily living (ADL)?

Population and setting

The population used to develop the rule consisted of independently living members of a community-based intervention called "Project Safety" in New Haven, Connecticut. Follow-up data were available for about 80% of subjects. The mean age was 79 years; 74% were female; and 84% were white. A similar group was used to validate the rule; their mean age was 78 years; 64% were female; and 79% were white.

Study size

The training group had 775 patients and the validation group 1038.

Pretest probability

Of the validation group, 18.4% developed ADL dependence during the 2.5-year follow-up.

Type of validation

Grade I: The test set was from a distinct population. The rule was developed in one group of patients and validated in another.

Comments

This rule was well validated in an appropriate setting, namely the community. It provides prognostic information for patients and their families and is quite simple to administer in the office setting.

Reference

Gill TM, Williams CS, Richardson ED, et al. A predictive model for ADL dependence in community-living older adults based on a reduced set of cognitive status items. J Am Geriatr Soc 1997;45:441–445.

CLINICAL PREDICTION RULE

1. Determine whether the patient is impaired regarding memory, orientation, both, or neither.

Memory: Ask the patient to remember three common items, such as pencil, coat and airplane. After the patient has done so, ask the orientation questions (below). Afterward, ask the patient to recall the items. A patient's memory is impaired if he or she fails to recall any of the three items.

Orientation: Ask the patient the following items:
1. What is the year?
2. What is the month?
3. What is your address?
4. What are the two main streets nearest your home?

A patient answering one or more of the above items incorrectly has impaired orientation.

2. Estimate the likelihood of ADL dependence.

No. of impaired domains	No. with ADL dependence/total	Relative risk
0	123/807 (15%)	1.0
1	39/151 (26%)	1.7 (1.2–2.3)
2	17/38 (45%)	3.0 (2.0–4.3)

Identification of Treatable Causes of Dementia

Clinical question

Which patients have a potentially treatable cause of dementia detectable by computed tomography (CT)?

Population and setting

Patients referred to a university geriatrics center for evaluation of cognitive impairment were included. Of 368 possible subjects, 20 were not demented and 144 did not undergo a complete evaluation.

Study size

The validation group had 204 patients.

Pretest probability

Of these patients, 4% had potentially treatable lesions: four tumors, one subdural hematoma, one intracerebral hematoma, and two with normal-pressure hydrocephalus. The mean age was 76 years; 70% were female. The mean Mini-Mental State score was 15.6 (out of 30).

Type of validation

Grade I: The validation group was from a distinct population. The rule was developed in one group of patients and validated in another.

Comments

This clinical rule gives some guidance as to whether an imaging study is needed for evaluation of dementia. Note, though, that the rule is not perfect, and some patients with a treatable cause of dementia were missed.

Reference

Martin DC, Miller J, Kapoor W, Karpf M, Boller F. Clinical prediction rules for computed tomographic scanning in senile dementia. Arch Intern Med 1987;147:77–80.

CLINICAL PREDICTION RULE

1. Patients meeting all of the following criteria do not need a head CT scan.

   Dementia present >1 month
   No head trauma during preceding week
   Gradual onset (>48 hours)
   No history of cerebrovascular accident
   No history of seizures
   No history of urinary incontinence
   No focal neurologic signs
   No papilledema
   No visual field defects
   No apraxia/ataxia of gait
   No headache

2. Interpretation: The rule identified 87.5% of patients with a treatable lesion (87.5% sensitivity, 37.2% specificity).

Determining the Cause of Dementia

Clinical question

What is the diagnosis of a patient presenting with dementia?

Population and setting

Consecutive patients seen in a Veterans Administration (VA) dementia clinic were included. The mean age was 72 years for patients with Alzheimer's disease, 70 years for those with multi-infarct dementia, and 54 years for those with other diagnoses; only 15% were female.

Study size

The validation group had 162 patients.

Pretest probability

Of the 162 patients, 92 had Alzheimer's, 42 multiinfarct dementia, and 27 another cause of dementia.

Type of validation

Grade I: The validation group was from a distinct population. The rule was developed in one group of patients and validated in another.

Comments

This clinical rule combines two rules: one to diagnose Alzheimer's and one to diagnose multiinfarct dementia. The validation is excellent, using a totally independent group of patients. Some of the variables are a little ambiguous, such as "emotional lability" and "relative preservation of personality."

Reference

Absher JR, Sultzer DL, Mahler ME, Fishman J. pC analysis facilitates dementia diagnosis. Med Decis Mak 1994;14:393–402.

CLINICAL PREDICTION RULE

1. First, calculate the Hachinski Ischemic Score by adding up the points for your patient.

Risk factor	Points
Abrupt onset	2
Stepwise deterioration	1
Fluctuating course	2
Nocturnal confusion	1
Relative preservation of personality	1
Depression	1
Somatic complaints	1
Emotional lability	1
Hypertension	2
History of stroke	2
Focal neurologic symptoms	2
Focal neurologic signs	2
Other signs of arteriosclerosis	1
Total:	

2. Interpretation: A Hachinski Ischemic Score ≥5 is consistent with multiinfarct dementia. If the Hachinski Ischemic Score is <5, add up the number of points in the Dementia of the Alzheimer's Type Inventory below.

3. Calculate the Dementia of the Alzheimer's Type Inventory by adding the points for your patient.

Risk factor	Points
Memory	
Normal or cue-responsive	0
Recalls 1 or 2 of 3 words, incomplete cueing	1
Disoriented, unable to learn 3 words, recall not aided by prompting	2
Visuospatial	
Normal or clumsy	0
Flattening, omissions, distortions	1
Disorganized or unrecognizable copies	2
Cognition	
Normal or impaired on complex abstractions/ calculations	0
Fails to abstract, difficulty with math	1
Fails to interpret simple proverbs or idioms, acalculia	2
Personality	
Disinhibition or depression	0
Appropriate insight	1
Unaware, indifferent, or irritable	2
Language	
Normal	0
Anomia, mild comprehension defects	1
Fluent aphasia with anomia, poor comprehension, paraphasia	2
Speech	
Mute, dysarthric	0
Slurred, amelodic, hypophonic	1
Normal	2
Psychomotor speed	
Slow, long latency	0
Hesitant	1
Normal, prompt responses	2
Posture	
Abnormal, flexed, extended, or distorted	0
Stooped or mild distortion	1
Normal, erect	2
Gait	
Hemiparetic, ataxic, apractic, or hyperkinetic	0
Shuffling, dyskinetic	1
Normal	2
Movements	
Tremor, akinesia, rigidity, or chorea	0
Imprecise, poorly coordinated	1
Normal	2
Total:	

4. Interpretation: If the Hachinski Ischemic Score <5:

Dementia of the Alzheimer's Type Inventory >10 is consistent with Alzheimer's dementia.

Dementia of the Alzheimer's Type Inventory ≤ 10 is consistent with other types of dementia syndromes.

Mini-Mental State Test for Diagnosis of Dementia

Clinical question

Is this patient demented?

Population and setting

Patients in the original study consisted of three groups. The first group was 69 patients chosen as clear examples of clinical conditions (dementia and affective disorders). The second group was 63 normal, elderly patients without evidence of cognitive impairment. The third group consisted of 137 consecutive patients with psychiatric admissions, of whom 9 were demented, 45 depressed, 24 schizophrenic, and 59 with drug abuse. In all three groups, 47% were male, and the mean age was 55 years. The mean age for demented patients was 76 years.

In a second, larger, prospective validation set in Italy, a new set of norms were developed based on a community-dwelling sample of the elderly. These new norms were then evaluated in a separate group.

Study size

The validation group in the original study had 269 patients, and the Italian validation study had 912 patients.

Pretest probability

Of 269 patients, 38 (14.1%) were demented in the original study and 40 of 912 (4.3%) in the Italian community-based validation.

Type of validation

Grade I: The validation group was from a distinct population. The rule was developed in one group of patients and validated in another.

Comments

Folstein et al.'s original description of the Mini-Mental State was prospective, but only half of the sample were consecutive patients; all were inpatients. A much more representative group of patients was studied by Grigoletto et al. The only question is of generalizability from Italy to the United States, although the results have good face validity.

References

Folstein M, Folstein SE, McHugh PR. "Mini Mental State": a practical method for grading the cognitive state of patients for the clinician. J Psychiatr Res 1975;12:129–198.

Grigoletto F, Zappala G, Anderson D, Lebowitz B. Norms for the Mini-Mental State Examination in a healthy population. Neurology 1999;53:315–320.

CLINICAL PREDICTION RULE

1. Calculate the patient's score.

Maximum score	Patient score	Question
5		What is the (year) (season) (date) (day) (month)?
5		Where are we: (state) (county) (town) (hospital) (floor)?
3		Name three objects: 1 second to say each. Then ask the patient to name all three. Give 1 point for each correct answer. Repeat them until he or she learns all 3. Count trials and record. Number of trials: ___________
5		Serial 7's: 1 point for each correct answer. Stop after 5 answers. Alternatively, spell "world" backward.
3		Ask for the three objects repeated above. Give 1 point for each correct answer.
2		Hold up a pencil and watch and ask the patient what each is.
1		Repeat the following: "No ifs, ands, or buts."
3		Follow a three-stage command: "Take a paper in your right hand, fold it in half, and put it on the floor."
1		Have the patient read and obey the following statement: "Close your eyes."
1		Write a sentence.
1		Copy a design (below).
30		

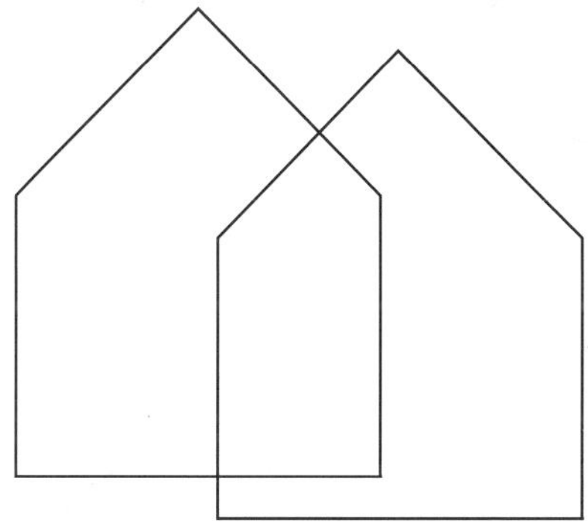

2. Interpret the Mini-Mental State (original study data).

Diagnosis	No. of patients	Mean score	Range
Dementia	38	10.2	0–22
Depression	71	24.6	8–30
Mania	14	26.6	20–30
Schizophrenia	24	24.6	1–30
Personality disorder with drug abuse	32	26.8	19–30
Neurosis	27	27.6	21–30
Normal	63	27.6	24–30

A Mini-Mental State (MMS) score <23 discriminates well between demented and normal patients.

3. Interpret the Mini-Mental State (Italian validation of MMS as a screening test). These are age-, gender-, and education-based normal values.

Education	Age (years)	Lower limit of normal
Men		
>10 Years	<77	27
	≥77	26
6–10 years	<54	26
	≥54	25
0–5 Years	<23	24
	23–43	23
	44–58	22
	59–71	21
	≥72	20
Women		
>10 Years	<34	28
	34–50	27
	≥51	26
6–10 Years	<29	27
	29–45	26
	46–61	25
	≥62	24
0–5 Years	<31	25
	31–44	24
	45–50	23
	51–55	22
	56–59	21
	60–64	20
	65–69	19
	70–73	18
	≥74	17

A score less than or equal to the lower limit of normal for a patient with the gender, age, and educational level above is an "abnormal" test.

4. An abnormal MMS is 85% sensitive and 89% specific. The corresponding likelihood ratios are 7.7 for a positive test and 0.17 for a negative test. The predictive values for different pretest probabilities of dementia are shown below.

Pretest probability	Probability of dementia given a positive test	Probability of dementia given a negative test
4% (Italian study)	24.4%	0.7%
8%	40.2%	1.4%
12%	51.3%	2.2%

"Time and Change" Test for Dementia

Clinical question

Is this patient demented?

Population and setting

Patients at the outpatient general medicine clinic of a university hospital were screened. The reference standard was a combination of the Blessed Dementia Rating Scale and the Mini-Mental State test. All patients were 70 years or older, with a mean age of 82; 67% were women.

Study size

Altogether, 100 patients were studied.

Pretest probability

Of these patients, 16% were demented.

Type of validation

Grade I: The test set was from a distinct population. The rule was developed in one group of patients and validated in another.

Comments

This is a quick and easy test to screen for dementia. Because the reference standard was itself a screening test, the accuracy as reported is somewhat inflated. The study did a good job of evaluating the reliability of the screening test and found that it is highly reproducible by different observers. Note that adding a time limit increases the sensitivity quite a bit.

Reference

Froehlich TE, Robison JT, Inouye SK. Screening for dementia in the outpatient setting: the time and change test. J Am Geriatr Soc 1998;46:1506–1511.

CLINICAL PREDICTION RULE

1. Perform the time and change test.

   Telling time: For the telling time task, the patient must respond to a clock face set at 11:10. Time to response is measured with a stopwatch. The patient is allowed two tries for a correct response within a 60-second period.

   Making change: For the making change task, three quarters, seven dimes, and seven nickels are placed in front of the patient. The participant is cued to give one dollar in change. Response time is measured with a stopwatch. The patient is allowed two tries within a 120-second period.

   Failure or an incorrect response to either task is a "positive" screening test for dementia.

2. Results of the test (untimed): Of the demented patients, 63% had an abnormal test (sensitivity); 96% of nondemented patients had a normal test (specificity).

3. Timed test interpretation: Reducing the time limit for each task improves sensitivity and worsens specificity.

   Time limits
   Telling time: ≤3 seconds
   Making change: ≤12 seconds

   All of the demented patients failed the timed "telling time" task, and 94% failed the timed "making change task." However, 63% of nondemented patients also failed the telling time task, and 54% failed the making change task.

■ SYNCOPE

Risk Stratification in Syncope

Clinical question

Which patients presenting with syncope are at risk for arrhythmias or death?

Population and setting

Adult patients presenting to an urban university medical center emergency department with a chief complaint of syncope were included. Syncope was defined as a sudden transient loss of consciousness associated with an inability to maintain postural tone that was not compatible with a seizure disorder, vertigo, dizziness (lightheadedness without loss of consciousness), coma, shock, or other states of altered consciousness. The mean age was 57 years (range 15–94 years); 54% were female; 23% were nonwhite.

Study size

The training group included 252 patients and the validation group 374.

Pretest probability

Of the patients in the validation group, 4.4% experienced an arrhythmia or death.

Type of validation

Grade II: The validation group was a separate sample from the same population, with data for the validation group gathered prospectively.

Comments

This well designed rule can help identify syncopal patients at high risk for morbidity and mortality. It was well validated and is quite easy to apply in the emergency room setting.

Reference

Martin TP, Hanusa BH, Kapoor WN. Risk stratification of patients with syncope. Ann Emerg Med 1997;29:459–466.

CLINICAL PREDICTION RULE

1. Count the number of the following risk factors your patient has.

Risk factor	Points
Abnormal ECG	1
History of ventricular arrhythmia	1
History of congestive heart failure	1
Age > 45 years	1
Total:	

2. Determine your patient's risk class and likelihood of morbidity and mortality in the table below.

Risk factors	Broadly defined cardiac arrhythmia[a]	Strictly defined cardiac arrhythmia[b]	Died within a year	Died of a cardiac cause within a year
0	3.3%	0%	1.1%	0%
1	6.0%	6.0%	8.5%	1.5%
2	17.0%	12.5%	16.0%	5.5%
3 or 4	45.5%	18.2%	27.3%	15.1%

[a]Broad definition of arrhythmia = ventricular tachycardia (VT) of three or more beats; symptomatic sinus pauses of 2 seconds or longer; symptomatic sinus bradycardia; supraventricular tachycardia (SVT) with symptoms or associated hypotension [systolic blood pressure (SBP) < 90 mm Hg]; atrial fibrillation with slow ventricular response (RR interval > 3 seconds); complete atrioventricular (AV) block; Mobitz II AV block; or evidence of pacemaker malfunction.

[b]Strict definition of arrhythmia = symptomatic or sustained VT (duration > 30 seconds or 100 beats), symptomatic SVT, symptomatic bradycardia, pauses of longer than 3 seconds, atrial fibrillation with slow ventricular response (RR interval > 3.0 seconds), complete AV block, Mobitz II AV block, or pacemaker malfunction.

■ ATTENTION DEFICIT HYPERACTIVITY DISORDER

Wender Utah Rating Scale for ADHD in Adults

Clinical question

Does this adult have a childhood history of attention deficit hyperactivity disorder (ADHD)?

Population and setting

The score was validated in a group of 81 adults with ADHD, 100 normal adults, and 70 adults with unipolar depression.

Study size

The validation group had 251 patients.

Pretest probability

This artificially created group had a 32% probability of ADHD.

Type of validation

Grade I: The validation group was from a distinct population. The rule was developed de novo and validated in a mixed population of patients.

Comments

This somewhat long and complicated score can help identify adults with ADHD.

Reference

Ward MF, Wender PH, Reimherr FW. The Wender Utah Rating Scale: an aid in the retrospective diagnosis of childhood attention deficit disorder. Am J Psychiatry 1993;150:885–890.

CLINICAL PREDICTION RULE

1. Add up the points for your patient.

Item	Not at all or very slightly	Mildly	Moderately	Quite a bit	Very much	Points for your patient
As a child I was (or had):						
Concentration problems, easily distracted	0	1	2	3	4	
Anxious, worrying	0	1	2	3	4	
Nervous, fidgety	0	1	2	3	4	
Inattentive, daydreaming	0	1	2	3	4	
Hot- or short-tempered, low boiling point	0	1	2	3	4	
Temper outbursts, tantrums	0	1	2	3	4	
Trouble with stick-to-it-iveness, not following through, failing to finish things started	0	1	2	3	4	
Stubborn, strong-willed	0	1	2	3	4	
Sad or blue, depressed, unhappy	0	1	2	3	4	
Disobedient with parents, rebellious, sassy	0	1	2	3	4	
Low opinion of myself	0	1	2	3	4	
Irritable	0	1	2	3	4	
Moody, ups and downs	0	1	2	3	4	
Angry	0	1	2	3	4	
Acting without thinking, impulsive	0	1	2	3	4	
Tendency to be immature	0	1	2	3	4	
Guilty feelings, regretful	0	1	2	3	4	
Losing control of myself	0	1	2	3	4	
Tendency to be or act irrational	0	1	2	3	4	
Unpopular with other children, did not keep friends for long, did not get along with other children	0	1	2	3	4	
Trouble seeing things from someone else's point of view	0	1	2	3	4	
Trouble with authorities, trouble with school, visits to principal's office	0	1	2	3	4	
Overall, a poor student, slow learner	0	1	2	3	4	
Trouble with mathematics or numbers	0	1	2	3	4	
Not achieving up to potential	0	1	2	3	4	
					Total:	

2. The score ranges from 0 to 100 points. A score of $\geq$ 36 correctly identifies 96% of adults with ADHD (96% sensitive); a score $<$ 36 correctly identifies 96% of the normal subjects (96% specific).

■ ALCOHOLISM

Detecting At-risk Drinking During Pregnancy (Poor, Urban Population)

Clinical question

Which women presenting for prenatal care display "risky drinking" behavior?

Population and setting

Adult women making their first visit to an inner city prenatal clinic were screened. All were African American and had low socioeconomic status. Mean age was 25 years.

Study size

Altogether, 2717 patients were studied to validate the rules.

Pretest probability

Based on a detailed interview, 181 of 2717 (6.7%) patients were "at risk drinkers."

Type of validation

Grade I: The test set was from a distinct population. The rule was developed in one group of patients and validated in another.

Comments

This was a well designed study, with the only limitation being the ability to generalize these results to all pregnant patients. However, the results should be highly generalizable to low income, African American women. Note that a positive CAGE test is useful, but a negative CAGE test is not good for ruling out at-risk drinking.

Reference

Russell M, Martier SS, Sokol RJ, et al. Detecting risk drinking during pregnancy: a comparison of four screening questionnaires. Am J Public Health 1996;86:1435–1439.

CLINICAL PREDICTION RULE

1. Calculate the patient's T-ACE (*t*olerance to alcohol, *a*nnoyed at criticism, *c*ut down on drinking, need an *e*ye-opener) score.

Item	Points
How many drinks can you hold? (positive = 6 or more)	2
Have you ever had a drink first thing in the morning to steady your nerves or get rid of a hangover?	1
Have you ever felt you ought to cut down on your drinking?	1
Have people annoyed you by criticizing your drinking?	1
Total:	

2. Calculate the TWEAK (*t*olerance, *w*orry, *e*ye-opener, *a*wakened, *K*ut down) score.

Item	Points
How many drinks can you hold? (positive = 6 or more)	2
Does your spouse (or do your parents) ever worry or complain about your drinking?	2
Have you ever had a drink first thing in the morning to steady your nerves or get rid of a hangover?	1
Have you ever awakened the morning after some drinking the night before and found that you could not remember a part of the evening before?	1
Have you ever felt you ought to cut down on your drinking?	1
Total:	

3. Calculate the CAGE (*c*ut down, *a*nnoyed by criticism, *g*uilty about drinking, *e*ye-opener drinks) score.

Item	Points
Have you ever felt you should cut down on your drinking?	1
Have people annoyed you by criticizing your drinking?	1
Have you ever felt bad or guilty about your drinking?	1
Have you ever had a drink first thing in the morning to steady your nerves or get rid of a hangover (eye-opener)?	1
Total:	

4. Interpret the T-ACE, TWEAK, and CAGE scores (a score ≥ 2 is considered positive).

Score	Sensitivity (%)	Specificity (%)	LR^+	LR^-	PV^+
TWEAK	91	77	4.0	0.1	22
T-ACE	88	79	4.2	0.2	23
CAGE	46	93	6.6	0.6	32

LR^+, LR^- = positive and negative likelihood ratios; PV^+ = positive predictive value for a pretest probability of 6.6%.

AUDIT Score for At-risk Drinking in the Primary Care Setting

Clinical question

Is the Alcohol Use Disorders Identification Test (AUDIT) score a useful screen for at-risk drinking in primary care?

Population and setting

Adult patients at a university-affiliated family practice center in Galveston, Texas were sampled. The refusal rate was less than 6%. Harmful use and dependence were defined based on a detailed interview using ICD-10 criteria. The average age was 39–47 years depending on the ethnic group, and women were deliberately oversampled in a 2:1 ratio owing to their lower risk of alcohol disorders.

Study size

Altogether, 1333 were used to validate the clinical rule.

Pretest probability

Of the subjects, 9% were hazardous alcohol users, and 6% were dependent.

Type of validation

Grade I: The test set was from a distinct population. The rule was developed in one group of patients and validated in another.

Comments

This is a well designed validation in a community setting. It demonstrates that the AUDIT is accurate for a variety of ethnic groups in the primary care setting.

Reference

Volk RJ, Steinbauer JR, Cantor SB, Holzer CE. The Alcohol Use Disorders Identification Test (AUDIT) as a screen for at-risk drinking in primary care patients of different racial/ethnic backgrounds. Addiction 1997;92:197–206.

CLINICAL PREDICTION RULE

1. Calculate the patient's AUDIT score. "The following questions pertain to your use of alcoholic beverages during the past year. A "drink" refers to a can or bottle of beer, a glass of wine, a wine cooler, or one cocktail or shot of hard liquor."

Item	Points
How often do you have a drink containing alcohol	
Never	0
Once a month or less	1
2–4 Times/month	2
2–3 Times/week	3
≥ 4 Times/week	4
How many drinks containing alcohol do you have on a typical day when you are drinking?	
1–2	0
3–4	1
5–6	2
7–9	3
≥10	4
How often do you have six or more drinks on one occasion?	
Never	0
Less than once a month	1
Monthly	2
Weekly	3
Daily or almost daily	4
How often during the last year have you found that you were not able to stop drinking once you had started?	
Never	0
Less than once a month	1
Monthly	2
Weekly	3
Daily or almost daily	4
How often during the last year have you failed to do what was normally expected from you because of drinking?	
Never	0
Less than once a month	1
Monthly	2
Weekly	3
Daily or almost daily	4
How often during the last year have you needed a first drink in the morning to get yourself going after a heavy drinking session?	
Never	0
Less than once a month	1
Monthly	2
Weekly	3
Daily or almost daily	4

Item	Points
How often during the last year have you had a feeling of guilt or remorse after drinking?	
Never	0
Less than once a month	1
Monthly	2
Weekly	3
Daily or almost daily	4
How often during the last year have you been unable to remember what happened the night before because you were drinking?	
Never	0
Less than once a month	1
Monthly	2
Weekly	3
Daily or almost daily	4
Have you or someone else been injured as a result of your drinking?	
No	0
Yes, but not in the past year	2
Yes, during the past year	4
Has a relative, friend, doctor, or other health care worker been concerned about your drinking or suggested you cut down?	
No	0
Yes, but not in the past year	2
Yes, during the past year	4
Total:	

2. Interpret the AUDIT score: The area under the receiver-operating characteristic (ROC) curve ranged from 0.896 for Mexican American men to 0.957 for white women. It performed similarly in different ethnic groups.

					Probability of at-risk drinking given this pretest probability		
AUDIT score	Sensitivity	Specificity	LR^+	LR^-	5%	10%	20%
≥4	85%	84%	5.3	0.57	22%	37%	57%
≥6	69%	93%	9.9	0.52	34%	52%	71%
≥8	51%	96%	12.8	0.50	40%	59%	76%
≥10	37%	98%	18.5	0.49	49%	67%	82%

At-risk drinking = problem alcohol users, hazardous alcohol users, and patients meeting ICD-10 criteria for alcohol dependence.

Detecting "Harmful Drinking" and Alcohol Dependence in the Emergency Department

Clinical question

Which patients presenting to the emergency department suffer from "harmful drinking" behavior, alcohol dependence, or both?

Population and setting

Adult patients presenting to the emergency department at the University of Mississippi Medical Center during a 6-month period were sampled. Those refusing (3%), those who left against medical advice (2%), and those who could not be interviewed (6%) were excluded. Breath alcohol tests were obtained from all participants, and a detailed interview based on the ICD-10 criteria was the gold standard.

Study size

The clinical rules were validated in 1330 patients.

Pretest probability

Altogether, 17% met ICD-10 criteria for harmful drinking and 19% for alcohol dependence.

Type of validation

Grade I: The test set was from a distinct population. The rule was developed in one group of patients and validated in another.

Comments

This was a well designed prospective validation of several clinical prediction rules.

Reference

Cherpitel CJ. Screening for alcohol problems in the emergency department. Ann Emerg Med 1995;26:158–166.

CLINICAL PREDICTION RULE

1. Calculate the patient's History of Trauma Scale score.

Item	Points
Since your 18th birthday, have you:	
Had any fractures or dislocations of bones or joints	1
Been injured in a traffic accident	1
Been injured in a fight or assault	1
Been injured after drinking	1
Injured your head	1
Total:	

2. Calculate the TWEAK score.

Item	Points
How many drinks can you hold? (positive = 6 or more)	2
Does your spouse (or do your parents) ever worry or complain about your drinking?	2
Have you ever had a drink first thing in the morning to steady your nerves or get rid of a hangover?	1
Have you ever awakened the morning after some drinking the night before and found that you could not remember a part of the evening before?	1
Have you ever felt you ought to cut down on your drinking?	1
Total:	

3. Calculate the CAGE score.

Item	Points
Have you ever felt that you should cut down on your drinking?	1
Have people annoyed you by criticizing your drinking?	1
Have you ever felt bad or guilty about your drinking?	1
Have you ever had a drink first thing in the morning to steady your nerves or get rid of a hangover (eye-opener)?	1
Total:	

4. Interpret the History of Trauma Scale, TWEAK score, and CAGE score.

					Positive predictive value for each pretest probability			
Score	Sensitivity	Specificity	LR+	LR−	5%	10%	20%	AUC
Prediction of current harmful drinking								
History of Trauma Score ≥ 2	52%	86%	3.7	0.6	16%	29%	48%	0.59
TWEAK ≥ 3	87%	86%	6.2	0.2	25%	41%	61%	0.91
CAGE ≥ 2	75%	88%	6.3	0.3	25%	41%	61%	0.84
Breath alcohol analysis positive	20%	94%	3.3	0.9	15%	27%	45%	NA
Prediction of alcohol dependence								
History of Trauma Score ≥ 2	49%	86%	3.5	0.6	16%	28%	47%	0.57
TWEAK ≥ 3	84%	86%	6.0	0.6	24%	40%	60%	0.89
CAGE ≥ 2	76%	90%	7.6	0.5	29%	46%	66%	0.85
Breath alcohol analysis positive	20%	94%	3.3	0.5	15%	27%	45%	NA

AUC = area under the receiver-operating characteristic curve; 0.5 = worthless test; 1.0 = perfect test; LR+, LR− = positive and negative likelihood ratios.

CAGE Score (in the Elderly)

Clinical question

Is this elderly patient an alcoholic?

Population and setting

A nonconsecutive sample of outpatients over age 60 years were included in the study. The study took place at an ambulatory medicine clinic at the Medical College of Virginia.

Study size

Altogether, 323 patients were studied.

Pretest probability

Of these patients, 33% met DSM-III criteria for a history of drinking problems, including alcohol abuse, dependence, or problem drinking.

Type of validation

Grade I: The validation group was from a distinct population. The rule was developed in one group of patients and validated in another.

Comments

This was an independent validation of the CAGE score in older patients. The area under the ROC curve was 0.862, consistent with an excellent ability to discriminate between problem drinkers and those without an alcohol problem. It is important to note that although 33% reported a history of a problem, only 6% reported a current alcohol problem; the other 27% reported that their problem was in remission. For example, a question in the CAGE could be answered in the positive because of a habit of eye-openers 30 years ago. It is not uncommon for problem drinking to "burn out" as a patient matures, although in other patients problem drinking may first arise during the later years. The CAGE should be considered a screening test, with the physician following up with a more detailed set of questions if the screen is positive.

Reference

Buchsbaum DG, Buchanan RG, Welsh J, Centor RM, Schnoll SH. Screening for drinking disorders in the elderly using the CAGE questionnaire. J Am Geriatr Soc 1992;40:662–665.

CLINICAL PREDICTION RULE

1. Calculate the patient's CAGE score.

Item	Points
Have you ever felt that you should cut down on your drinking?	1
Have people annoyed you by criticizing your drinking?	1
Have you ever felt bad or guilty about your drinking?	1
Have you ever had a drink first thing in the morning to steady your nerves or get rid of a hangover (eye-opener)?	1
Total:	

2. Determine the probability of a history of alcoholism or problem drinking based on the patient's CAGE score and the prevalence of drinking problems in this population.

	Prevalence of drinking problems in this population				
CAGE score	3%	5%	10%	15%	20%
0	3%	5%	10%	15%	20%
1	11%	17%	30%	41%	49%
2	19%	28%	46%	57%	66%
3	23%	33%	51%	63%	70%
4	48%	61%	77%	84%	88%

Heavy Use of Alcohol by the General Population

Clinical question

Which patients in a general population survey are heavy consumers of alcohol?

Population and setting

All men between the ages of 45 and 59 participating in a collaborative heart study in two British towns were included. This constitutes 90% of the potential population in these two towns.

Study size

The training group had 2512 patients and the validation group 2348.

Pretest probability

"Heavy alcohol use" was defined as the upper 10% of self-reported alcohol use and was therefore present in 10% of patients.

Type of validation

Grade I: The validation group was from a distinct population. The rule was developed in one group of patients and validated in another.

Comments

The major issue here is one of generalizability, given the differences in social milieu and "pub life" between Britain and other countries, especially the United States. On the other hand, the predictor variables are also highly objective, so it is likely that this rule can be used in other populations.

Reference

Lichtenstein MJ, Burger MC, Yamell JW, et al. Derivation and validation of a prediction rule for identifying heavy consumers of alcohol. Alcohol Clin Exp Res 1989;13: 626–630.

CLINICAL PREDICTION RULE

1. Calculate the patient's risk score.

   Definitions

   MCV = mean corpuscular volume
   TG = triglyceride
   SBP = systolic blood pressure (mm Hg)
   BMI = body mass index (kg/m^2)
   HDL = high density lipoprotein cholesterol (mg/dl)

$$\text{Risk score} = \text{MCV} + (\text{BMI} \times 0.31) + (\text{SBP} \times 0.08) + (\text{HDL} \times 9.24) + (\text{TG} \times 2.2)$$

Risk Score	No. with low consumption (0–525 ml/week)	With high consumption (>526 ml/week)	Likelihood ratio for high consumption
0–120.04	429	7%	0.06
120.05–123.34	428	17%	0.4
123.35–126.22	420	31%	1.2
126.23–129.95	388	50%	1.2
129.96–132.89	174	47%	2.4
132.90–136.29	79	30%	2.4
>136.30	68	40%	7.4

DEPRESSION AND ANXIETY

Primary Care Evaluation of Medical Disorders (PRIME-MD) Screening Instrument (Self-administered Version)

Clinical question

Is this patient at risk for depression or anxiety?

Population and setting

This study took place in the offices of 21 general internists and 41 family physicians. The mean age was 46 years (range 19–99 years); 66% were female; 79% were white.

Study size

Of 3000 patients screened, 585 had a psychiatric interview within 48 hours (the reference standard).

Pretest probability

Altogether, 29% had a psychiatric diagnosis.

Type of validation

Type I: The validation group came from a distinct group of patients.

Comments

The results reported here are for a self-administered survey. It is interesting that only 32% of the "new" diagnoses resulted in prescription of a drug or referral for counseling. This supports the contention of many primary care physicians that they see a somewhat different spectrum of depression than do psychiatrists. The disease is less clearly defined and often less disabling, and resistance to treatment may be high.

Reference

Spitzer RL, Kroenke K, Williams JB, et al. Validation and utility of a self-report version of PRIME-MD: the PHQ Primary Care Study. JAMA 1999;282:1737–1744.

CLINICAL PREDICTION RULE

1. Have the patient answer the following three questions.

1. Over the *last 2 weeks,* how often have you been bothered by the following symptoms?	Not at all	Several days	More than half the days	Nearly every day
a. Little interest or pleasure in doing things				
b. Feeling down, depressed, or hopeless				
c. Trouble falling or staying asleep, or sleeping too much				
d. Feeling tired or having little energy				
e. Poor appetite or overeating				
f. Feeling bad about yourself—or that you are a failure or have let yourself or your family down				
g. Trouble concentrating on things, such as reading the newspaper or watching television				
h. Moving or speaking so slowly that other people could have noticed? Or the opposite—being so fidgety or restless that you have been moving around a lot more than usual				
i. Thoughts that you would be better off dead or of hurting yourself in some way				

2. Questions about anxiety	Yes	No
a. In the *last 4 weeks,* have you had an anxiety attack—suddenly feeling fear or panic?		
If you checked "No", go to question 2.		
b. Has this ever happened before?		
c. Do some of these attacks come *suddenly out of the blue,* that is, in situations where you don't expect to be nervous or uncomfortable?		
d. Do these attacks bother you a lot or are you worried about having another attack?		
e. During your last bad anxiety attack, did you have symptoms such as shortness of breath, sweating, your heart racing or pounding, dizziness or faintness, tingling or numbness, nausea or upset stomach?		

3. If you checked off *any* problems on this questionnaire so far, how *difficult* have these problems made it for you to do your work, take care of things at home, or get along with other people:

Not difficult at all
Somewhat difficult
Very difficult
Extremely difficult

4. Interpret the score.

Major depressive syndrome: Answers to 1a or b and five or more of 1a–i are at least "More than half the days" (count 1i if present at all)

Other depressive syndrome: Answers to 1a or b and two, three, or four of 1a–i are at least "More than half the days" (count 1i if present at all)

Panic syndrome: Answers to 2a–e are "Yes"

The sensitivity, specificity, and likelihood ratios (positive and negative) of the self-administered PRIME-MD for these diagnoses compared with the psychiatric interview are shown below:

Diagnosis	Sensitivity	Specificity	LR^+	LR^-
Any PRIME-MD psychiatric diagnosis	75%	90%	7.5	0.3
Any mood disorder	61%	94%	10.2	0.4
Major depressive disorder	73%	98%	36.5	0.3
Any anxiety disorder	63%	97%	21.0	0.4
Panic disorder	81%	99%	81.0	0.2

Zung Self-Rating Depression Scale

Clinical question

Is this patient depressed?

Population and setting

The Zung Self-Rating Depression Scale was developed from a review of the literature and first tested on 56 patients admitted to a psychiatric facility with an initial diagnosis of depression.

Study size

The validation group had 56 patients

Pretest probability

Of the 56 patients, 31 had a discharge diagnosis of depression.

Type of validation

Grade IV: The training group was used as the validation group.

Comments

This widely used scale is probably more practical as a research tool than as an in-office screen for depression.

Reference

Zung WW. A self-rating depression scale. Arch Gen Psychiatry 1965;12:63–70.

CLINICAL PREDICTION RULE

1. Zung Depression Scale

Question	A little of the time	Some of the time	Good part of the time	Most of the time
1. I feel down-hearted and blue				
2. Morning is when I feel the best				
3. I have crying spells or feel like it				
4. I have trouble sleeping at night				
5. I eat as much as I used to				
6. I still enjoy sex				
7. I notice that I am losing weight				
8. I have trouble with constipation				
9. My heart beats faster than usual				
10. I get tired for no reason				
11. My mind is as clear as it used to be				
12. I find it easy to do the things I used to				
13. I am restless and can't keep still				
14. I feel hopeful about the future				
15. I am more irritable than usual				
16. I find it easy to make decisions				
17. I feel that I am useful and needed				
18. My life is pretty full				
19. I feel that others would be better off if I were dead				
20. I still enjoy the things I used to do				

2. Score the patient's responses as shown below (range 20 to 80).

Question	A little of the time	Some of the time	Good part of the time	Most of the time	Points
1. I feel down-hearted and blue	1	2	3	4	
2. Morning is when I feel the best	4	3	2	1	
3. I have crying spells or feel like it	1	2	3	4	
4. I have trouble sleeping at night	1	2	3	4	
5. I eat as much as I used to	4	3	2	1	
6. I still enjoy sex	4	3	2	1	
7. I notice that I am losing weight	1	2	3	4	
8. I have trouble with constipation	1	2	3	4	
9. My heart beats faster than usual	1	2	3	4	
10. I get tired for no reason	1	2	3	4	
11. My mind is as clear as it used to be	4	3	2	1	
12. I find it easy to do the things I used to	4	3	2	1	
13. I am restless and can't keep still	1	2	3	4	
14. I feel hopeful about the future	4	3	2	1	
15. I am more irritable than usual	1	2	3	4	
16. I find it easy to make decisions	4	3	2	1	
17. I feel that I am useful and needed	4	3	2	1	
18. My life is pretty full	4	3	2	1	
19. I feel that others would be better off if I were dead	1	2	3	4	
20. I still enjoy the things I used to do	4	3	2	1	
				Score:	

3. Interpret the score. Patients with a score ≥ 50 are likely to be depressed.

Two-Question Instrument for Depression Screening

Clinical question

Is this patient depressed?

Population and setting

Consecutive adult patients without mania or schizophrenia presenting to an urgent care clinic at the San Francisco VA Medical Center were studied. Not surprisingly, 97% were male. The average age was 53 years; 29% were African American; 8% were homeless; 86% had a high school education or higher; 53% had an annual income under $10,000; and 71% were not working.

Study size

Altogether, 536 patients were studied.

Pretest probability

Of the patients studied, 18% were depressed based on the reference test (Quick Diagnostic Interview Schedule).

Type of validation

Grade I: The validation group was from a distinct population. The rule was developed in one group of patients and validated in another. The two questions were selected based on the results of the PRIME-MD studies (see above).

Comments

This rule was well validated, but the generalizability nonmale populations and groups outside the urban poor population is questionable.

Reference

Whooley MA, Avins AL, Miranda J, Browner WS. Case-finding instruments for depression: two questions are as good as many. J Gen Intern Med 1997;12:439–445.

CLINICAL PREDICTION RULE

Ask your patient these two questions:

1. During the past month, have you often been bothered by feeling down, depressed, or hopeless?
2. During the past month, have you often been bothered by little interest or pleasure in doing things?

A positive response to either question identified 96% of depressed patients. The rule was 57% specific (of 100 patients identified as not depressed by the rule, 57% actually were not depressed).

Geriatric Depression Scale

Clinical question

Is this elderly patient depressed?

Population and setting

The scale was tested on a group of 20 nondepressed and 51 depressed elderly patients in the San Francisco Bay area.

Study size

The scale was validated in a group of 71 patients.

Pretest probability

This parameter is not applicable: this was a case-control validation.

Type of validation

Grade II: The test set was a separate sample from the same population, with data for the test set gathered prospectively.

Comments

This study is limited by the small size. In the study the Geriatric Depression Scale was better able to discriminate between depressed and nondepressed elders than the Zung or Hamilton scores.

Reference

Brink TL, Yesavage JA, Lum O, et al. Screening tests for geriatric depression. Clin Gerontol 1982;1:37–43.

CLINICAL PREDICTION RULE

1. Score 1 point for each depressive/abnormal answer. The scale is designed to be self-administered.

Question	Depressive answer	Points
1. Are you basically satisfied with your life?	No	1
2. Have you dropped many of your activities and interests?	Yes	1
3. Do you feel that your life is empty?	Yes	1
4. Do you often get bored?	Yes	1
5. Are you hopeful about the future?	No	1
6. Are you bothered by thoughts you can't get out of your head?	Yes	1
7. Are you in good spirits most of the time?	No	1
8. Are you afraid that something bad is going to happen to you?	No	1
9. Do you feel happy most of the time?	No	1
10. Do you often feel helpless?	Yes	1
11. Do you often get restless and fidgety?	Yes	1
12. Do you prefer to stay at home, rather than going out and doing new things?	Yes	1
13. Do you frequently worry about the future?	Yes	1
14. Do you feel you have more problems with memory than most?	Yes	1
15. Do you think it is wonderful to be alive now?	No	1
16. Do you often feel downhearted and blue?	Yes	1
17. Do you feel pretty worthless the way you are now?	Yes	1
18. Do you worry a lot about the past?	Yes	1
19. Do you find life very exciting?	No	1
20. Is it hard for you to get started on new projects?	Yes	1
21. Do you feel full of energy?	No	1
22. Do you feel that your situation is hopeless?	Yes	1
23. Do you think that most people are better off than you are?	Yes	1
24. Do you frequently get upset over little things?	Yes	1
25. Do you frequently feel like crying?	Yes	1
26. Do you have trouble concentrating?	Yes	1
27. Do you enjoy getting up in the morning?	No	1
28. Do you prefer to avoid social gatherings?	Yes	1
29. Is it easy for you to make decisions?	No	1
30. Is your mind as clear as it used to be?	No	1
	Total:	

2. A score of 0–10 is normal, and a score > 10 is a positive screen for depression. This test is 84% sensitive and 95% specific. Use the overall probability of depression in your setting and the table below to estimate the probability of depression given by the Geriatric Depression Score (GDS).

Overall rate of depression among elderly patients in your setting	Probability of depression	
	GDS 0–10	GDS > 10
10%	2%	65%
20%	4%	81%
30%	7%	88%

COMA

Likelihood of Bad Outcome for Nontraumatic Coma

Clinical question

What is the likelihood of death or severe disability in patients with nontraumatic coma?

Population and setting

Patients were included if they were described by a physician as comatose, unconscious, or obtunded and had a Glasgow Coma Score of 9 or less for 6 hours or more. Patients were excluded if trauma, drug intoxication, hypothermia, or an operative complication precipitated the coma or if they had one of the following metabolic causes of coma: diabetic ketotic coma, nonketotic hyperosmolar coma, thyrotoxicosis, myxedema coma, hepatic encephalopathy, coma attributed to uremia, coma due to hyponatremia or hypernatremia, or coma due to hypocalcemia or hypercalcemia. Patients with coma due to hypoglycemia or hypoxemia were included. Patients were not included if they died, were declared brain-dead, or left the hospital within 48 hours of admission. The mean age was 66 years in the validation group; 41% were over age 70; 55% were women. The most common causes of coma were cardiac arrest (29%), intracerebral hemorrhage (24%), cerebral infarct (17%), subarachnoid hemorrhage (12%), sepsis (10%), and central nervous system infection (6%).

Study size

The training group had 247 patients and the validation group 349.

Pretest probability

The 2-month mortality was 66% in the validation group; at 2 months another 23% were classified as severely disabled. Only 8% survived without severe disability at 2 months, and 3% had an unknown outcome.

Type of validation

Grade II: The validation group was a separate sample from the same population, with data for the validation group gathered prospectively.

Comments

This simple rule can help identify patients at high risk for death or severe disability. This important information can help families make more appropriate decisions about continuing care for their loved ones.

Reference

Hamel MB, Goldman L, Teno J, et al. Identification of comatose patients at high risk for death or severe disability. JAMA 1995;273:1842–1848.

CLINICAL PREDICTION RULE

Definitions
Abnormal brain stem response = Brain stem responses were defined as abnormal if a patient had one or more of the following: absent pupillary responses, absent corneal response, or absent or dysconjugate roving eye movements.
Absent verbal response = Patients who were intubated were considered to have "absent verbal response" if they were generally unresponsive.

1. Count the number of risk factors for your patient.

Risk factor	Points
Abnormal brain stem response	1
Absent verbal response	1
Absent withdrawal to pain	1
Creatinine level ≥ 1.5 mg/dl (132.6 μmol/L)	1
Age ≥ 70 years	1
Total:	

2. Determine their risk of death at 2 months based on the number of risk factors.

No. of risk factors	Mortality at 2 months (95% CI)
0	29% (15–46)
1	51% (38–63)
2	60% (50–71)
3	84% (73–91)
4	96% (87–100)
5	100% (66–100)

CI = confidence interval.

3. Prediction of death *or* severe disability at 2 months: If a patient had abnormal brain stem function or an absence of withdrawal response to pain, the rate of death or severe disability at 2 months was 97% (95% CI:93–99%).

■ DELIRIUM

Risk of Delirium after Elective Noncardiac Surgery

Clinical question

Which patients will experience delirium after elective noncardiac surgery?

Population and setting

Patients over age 50 admitted for major elective noncardiac surgery to the surgery and gynecology services at Brigham and Women's Hospital in Boston were included. The mean age was 68 years; 45% were male.

Study size

The training group had 876 patients and the validation group 465.

Pretest probability

Of the validation group, 8% developed delirium during the postoperative period.

Type of validation

Grade II: The validation group was a separate sample from the same population, with data for the validation group gathered prospectively.

Comments

This was a well designed rule that could be built into the standard preoperative evaluation of elderly patients to identify those at high risk for delirium. For those at high risk, special measures can be taken to prevent delirium.

References

Inouye SK, Bogardus ST, Charpentier PA, et al. A multicomponent intervention to prevent delirium in hospitalized older patients. N Engl J Med 1999;340:669–676.

Marcantonio ER, Goldman L, Manglone CM, et al. A clinical prediction rule for delirium after elective noncardiac surgery. JAMA 1994;271:134–139.

CLINICAL PREDICTION RULE

1. Add up the number of points by your patient.

Variable	Points
Age ≥ 70 years	1
Alcohol abuse	1
TICS score < 30[a]	1
Unable to walk 4 km/hr for one block, make their bed, or dress themselves without stopping	1
Na^+ < 130 or > 150 mEq/L *or* K^+ < 3.0 or > 6.0 mEq/L *or* Glucose < 60 or > 300 mg/dl	1
Aortic aneurysm surgery	2
Noncardiac thoracic surgery	1
Total:	

[a]Telephone Interview for Cognitive Status (Brandt J, Spencer M, Folstein MF. The telephone interview for cognitive status. Neuropsychiatry Neuropsychol Behav Neurol 1988;1:111–117).

2. Determine the risk of delirium based on the number of points.

Points	Likelihood of postoperative delirium
0	2%
1	8%
2	13%
>2	50%

Risk of Delirium in Hospitalized Medical Patients

Clinical question

Which patients on a medical ward will experience delirium?

Population and setting

Consecutive patients aged 70 years and older with no delirium at baseline were included. Patients who could not be interviewed (n = 147), who were discharged in less than 48 hours (n = 119), who were enrolled from a previous admission (n = 100), whose physician refused permission (n = 47), or who had other reasons such as respiratory isolation (n = 61) were excluded. The mean age was 78.5 years; 55% were female; and 91% were white.

Study size

The training group had 196 patients and the validation group 312.

Pretest probability

In all, 15% had new-onset delirium by the ninth hospital day.

Type of validation

Grade II: The validation group was a separate sample from the same population, with data for the validation group gathered prospectively.

Comments

This is a well designed clinical rule that is somewhat easier to apply than that described by Marcantonio et al. (see above). Some of the variables could be more carefully defined, such as "prolonged bleeding," but this is not a fatal flaw. This is the rule that was used in a later intervention study by the same author.

References

Inouye SK, Bogardus ST, Charpentier PA, et al. A multicomponent intervention to prevent delirium in hospitalized older patients. N Engl J Med 1999;340:669–676.

Inouye SK, Charpentier PA. Precipitating factors for delirium in hospitalized elderly persons: predictive model and interrelationship with baseline vulnerability. JAMA 1996;275:852–857.

CLINICAL PREDICTION RULE

1. Add up the number of points for your patient.

Variable	Points
Use of physical restraints	1
More than three medications added during hospitalization	1
Use of bladder catheter	1
Albumin < 3.0 g/dl	1
One or more of the following:	
ED stay > 12 hours	
Volume overload	
IV catheter complications	
Prolonged bleeding	
UTI following instrumentation	
Transfusion reaction	
Unintentional injury	
New pressure ulcer	1
Total:	

ED = emergency department; IV = intravenous; UTI = urinary tract infection.

2. Determine the risk of delirium based on the number of points.

Points	Delirium rate per person	Relative risk of new onset delirium	Delirium rate per day
0	4%	1.0	0.5%
1–2	20%	5.0	3.3%
3–5	35%	8.9	8.2%

13

Pediatrics

■ SEPSIS AND SERIOUS INFECTION

Meningococcal Disease

Clinical question

Which children with invasive meningococcal disease will have an adverse outcome?

Population and setting

Consecutive patients over a 5-year period under age 20 admitted with invasive meningococcal disease to one of three university hospitals were included. The mean age was 27 months; 52% were male.

Study size

The training group had 154 patients and the validation group 92.

Pretest probability

Altogether, 9% died and 3% had an amputation.

Type of validation

Grade I: The validation group was from a distinct population. The rule was developed in one group of patients and validated in another.

Comments

This is actually two clinical rules, each using a different combination of variables. Both are well validated.

Reference

Malley R, Huskins WC, Kupperman N. Multivariate predictive models for adverse outcome of invasive meningococcal disease in children. J Pediatr 1996;129:702–710.

CLINICAL PREDICTION RULE

Two models were developed using different variables. Results are reported for the validation group; the second model is smaller because fibrinogen levels were not measured in all patients.

Definitions

Low systolic blood pressure (SBP): 0–1 month, <70 mm Hg; 1 month to 5 years, <80 mm Hg; ≥5 years, <90 mm Hg

Poor perfusion: cool extremities, mottled skin, or capillary refill > 2 seconds, in association with low SBP

Model 1

1. Count the number of points for your patient.

Variable	Points
Absolute neutrophil count < 3000/mm^3	1
Poor perfusion	1
Platelet count < 150,000/mm^3	1
Total:	

2. Find your patient in the table below.

No. of points	Adverse outcomes/total in category
0	1/57 (1.8%)
1	1/15 (6.7%)
2	3/5 (60%)
3	6/6 (100%)

Model 2

1. Count the number of points for your patient.

Variable	Points
Fibrinogen < 2.5 g/L (250 mg/dl)	1
Absolute neutrophil count < 3000 mm^3	1
Total:	

2. Find your patient in the table below.

No. of points	Adverse outcomes/total in category
0	0/29
1	1/6 (16.7%)
2	8/9 (88.8%)

Rochester Criteria for Infants Under 2 Months with Fever

Clinical question

Which well-appearing children under 2 months of age who have a temperature >38°C have a serious bacterial infection?

Population and setting

Consecutive febrile patients under 60 days of age with a documented rectal temperature ≥38°C were included. They were excluded if complete data were not available ($n = 54$) or if they appeared ill ($n = 2$). The study took place in an emergency department and a pediatric clinic.

Study size

A total of 931 infants were studied, of whom 511 met low risk criteria.

Pretest probability

Of the 931 infants, 7.1% had bacteremia.

Type of validation

Grade I: The validation group was from a distinct population. The rule was developed in one group of patients and validated in another.

Comments

This is a well validated clinical rule. Only about 1% of the low risk infants had bacteremia, compared with more than 10% of the high-risk group. Other than a careful history and physical examination, only a complete blood count, urinalysis, and stool smear (if diarrhea) were needed.

Reference

Jaskiewica JA, McCarthy CA, Richardson AC, et al. Febrile infants at low risk for serious bacterial infections: an appraisal of the Rochester criteria and implications for management. Pediatrics 1994;94:390–396.

CLINICAL PREDICTION RULE

Patients are at low risk if they meet all of the following criteria.

1. Infant appears generally well
2. Infant has been previously healthy (all of the following are true)

   - Born at term (≥37 weeks' gestation)
   - Did not receive perinatal antimicrobial therapy
   - Was not treated for unexplained hyperbilirubinemia
   - Had not received and was not receiving antimicrobial agents
   - Had not been previously hospitalized
   - Had no chronic or underlying illness
   - Was not hospitalized longer than mother

3. No evidence of skin, soft tissue, bone, joint, or ear infection
4. Laboratory values (all of the following are true)

   - Peripheral blood white blood cell (WBC) count 5000–15,000 cells/mm^3
   - Absolute band form count ≤1500/mm^3
   - ≤10 WBCs per high power field (×40) on microscopic examination of centrifuged urine sediment
   - ≤5 WBCs per high power field (×40) on microscopic examination of a stool smear (only for infants with diarrhea)

Interpretation: The sensitivity is 92%, specificity 54%, positive likelihood ratio (LR^+) 2.0, and LR^- 0.15 for the identification of children with serious bacterial infection. In this study, low risk children had a 1.1% risk of serious bacterial infection (5/511). If at high risk, approximately 10% had a serious bacterial infection.

Yale Observation Score

Clinical question

What is the risk of bacteremic illness in febrile children 3–24 months of age?

Population and setting

The population studied included infants age 3–24 months with a temperature >39.4°C (102.9°F). Patients with recent antibiotic use or overt signs of meningitis or sepsis were excluded.

Study size

Altogether, 154 children were studied.

Pretest probability

Of these children, 12.3% had a bacteremic illness.

Type of validation

Grade I: The test set was from a distinct population. The rule was developed in one group of patients and validated in another.

Comments

The Yale Observation Score is somewhat less accurate and helpful than the Rochester Criteria. This validation gives information on how to interpret the score before and after fever reduction with acetaminophen in standard doses. Fever reduction reduces the sensitivity a lot, but increases specificity only a little. Overall usefulness as measured by the ratio of the positive and negative likelihood ratios (LR^+, LR^-) suggests that the score is best calculated before fever reduction.

Reference

Baker RC, Tiller T, Bausher JC, et al. Severity of disease correlated with fever reduction in febrile infants. Pediatrics 1989;83:1016–1019.

CLINICAL PREDICTION RULE

1. Add up the points for your patient.

Item	Points
Quality of cry	
Strong with normal tone or content and not crying	1
Whimpering or sobbing	3
Weak or moaning or high-pitched	5
Reaction to parent stimulation	
Cries briefly then stops or content and not crying	1
Cries off and on	3
Continual cry or hardly responds	5
State variation	
If awake, stays awake, or if asleep and stimulated wakes up quickly	1
Eyes close briefly and then awakens or awakens after prolonged stimulation	3
Falls to sleep or does not rouse	5
Color	
Pink	1
Pale extremities or acrocyanosis	3
Pale or cyanotic or mottled or ashen	5
Hydration	
Skin normal, eyes normal, mucous membranes moist	1
Skin and eyes normal and mouth slightly dry	3
Skin doughy or tented and dry mucous membranes and/or sunken eyes	5
Response (talk, smile) to social overtures	
Smiles or alerts (≤2 months)	1
Brief smile or alerts briefly (≤2 months)	3
No smile; face anxious, dull, expressionless, or no alerting (≤2 months)	5

2. Interpret the results below.

Parameter	Sensitivity	Specificity	LR^+	LR^-
Before fever reduction	68%	77%	3.0	0.4
After fever reduction	21%	92%	2.6	0.9

Syracuse Croup Score

Clinical question

Which children with croup are at high risk for requiring intubation?

Population and setting

This study took place at a Welsh university hospital that had a catchment with 80,000 children age 0–14 years. Only children who were admitted to the hospital were included in the follow-up.

Study size

Two validation phases were used, one with 165 children and one with 134 children.

Pretest probability

Of the patients assessed, 8% were admitted to the intensive care unit (ICU), and 2% were intubated.

Type of validation

Grade I: The validation group was from a distinct population. The rule was developed in one group of patients and validated in another.

Comments

This is a validation of the Syracuse Croup Score, showing that it had good predictive accuracy even when transported across the ocean to a very different setting. For the first phase of validation, children were admitted to the ICU based on clinical grounds and without knowledge of the croup score. No child with a score > 5 was admitted to the ICU or transferred there within 24 hours of admission. For the second phase, a cutoff of > 5 was used to guide admission to the ICU.

Reference

Shortland G, Warner J, Dearden A, Singh G, Tarpey J. Validation of a croup score and its use in triaging children with croup. Anesthesia 1994;49:903–906.

CLINICAL PREDICTION RULE

1. Calculate your patient's score.

Characteristic	0	1	2	3	Points
Stridor	None	Faintly audible	Easily audible		
Cyanosis	None	Minimal	Obvious		
Sternal retraction	None	Present			
Respiratory rate (breaths/minute)					
0–5 kg	<35	36–40	41–45	>45	
5.1–10 kg	<30	31–35	36–40	>40	
>10 kg	<20	21–24	25–30	>30	
Pulse rate (beats/minute)					
<3 months	< 150	150–165	166–190	>190	
3–6 months	<130	130–145	146–170	>170	
7–12 months	<120	120–135	136–150	>150	
1–3 years	<110	110–125	126–140	>140	
3–5 years	<90	91–100	101–120	>120	
				Total:	

2. Interpret the score: Children with a score >5 are at especially high risk of requiring intubation. In this study, only 2 of 123 children with an initial score ≤5 eventually required treatment in the ICU. Regular recalculation of the score with every shift is advised to track deterioration or improvement.

NEONATOLOGY

Optimal Endotracheal Tube Length in Infants

Clinical question

What is the appropriate length for an endotracheal tube in newborn infants?

Population and setting

Sick newborn infants at New York University Medical Center requiring intubation were included. In the training group, 66 infants were intubated using the oral route and 18 by the nasal route.

Study size

The training group had 84 patients and the validation group 50.

Pretest probability

This parameter is not applicable.

Type of validation

Grade II: The validation group was a separate sample from the same population, with data for the validation group gathered prospectively.

Comments

This simple rule should be posted in every delivery room.

Reference

Shukla HK, Hendricks-Munoz K, Atakent Y, Rapaport S. Rapid estimation of insertional length of endotracheal intubation in newborn infants. J Pediatr 1997;131:561–564.

CLINICAL PREDICTION RULE

Definitions
NTL = nasal tragus length (cm)
STL = sternal length (cm)

Route	Using NTL	Using STL
Orotracheal	NTL + 1 cm	STL + 1 cm
Nasotracheal	NTL + 2 cm	STL + 2 cm

The NTL may be preferred because STL measurement can interfere with auscultation of the heart.

Probability of Developing Symptomatic Patent Ductus Arteriosus

Clinical question

What is the likelihood that a low-birth-weight neonate will develop symptomatic patent ductus arteriosus (PDA)?

Population and setting

All infants weighing 1500 g or less at the Vanderbilt neonatal intensive care unit (NICU) who survived at least 72 hours were included in the study population.

Study size

The training group had 100 patients and the validation group 94.

Pretest probability

Of the validation group, 51% subsequently developed symptomatic PDA.

Type of validation

Grade II: The validation group was a separate sample from the same population, with data for the validation group gathered prospectively.

Comments

This small study provides guidance for identifying neonates with a high likelihood of PDA and who might benefit from more aggressive screening. Note the age of the study—it should be prospectively validated in your own setting before being applied clinically. This is particularly true of using it to *reduce* vigilance for PDA.

Reference

Cotton RB, Lindstrom DP, Stahlman MT. Early prediction of symptomatic patent ductus arteriosus from perinatal risk factors: a discriminant analysis model. Acta Paediatr Scand 1981;70:723.

CLINICAL PREDICTION RULE

1. Calculate the risk score.

Risk factor	Points if risk factor is present
Birth weight (g)	___ grams
Clinical hyaline membrane disease	−456
Distending airway pressure[a]	−220
Intrauterine growth retardation	+466
Acute perinatal stress[b]	−104
Total:	

[a]Use of distending airway pressure during the first 24 hours after birth, other than during resuscitation in the delivery room.

[b]Any of the following: Apgar score < 3 at 1 minute or <5 at 5 minutes or initial pH within 12 hours after birth < 7.20; initial central hematocrit < 45% or falling to <40% within 24 hours after birth; initial systolic blood pressure within 12 hours after birth < 40 mm Hg if birth weight > 1000 g or <35 mm Hg if birth weight < 1000 g; placenta previa with hemorrhage; placental abruption or breech delivery; umbilical cord prolapse; or vaginal bleeding within 24 hours before delivery.

Thus a child with a birth weight of 1246 g, who has no evidence of hyaline membrane disease, no use of distending airway pressure, but did have intrauterine growth retardation and acute perinatal stress would have a score of 1246 + 0 + 0 + 466 − 104 = 1608 points.

2. Interpret the score.

Score	No. of patients	% With PDA
≤852	59	74
>852	35	11

3. This corresponds to the following test characteristics.

Sensitivity: 92%
Specificity: 67%
Positive likelihood ratio (LR^+): 2.8
Negative likelihood ratio (LR^-): 0.12

Neonatal Outcome: Clinical Risk Index for Babies (CRIB) Score

Clinical question

What is the prognosis for premature and low-birth-weight infants in the neonatal intensive care unit?

Population and setting

All infants without an "inevitably lethal congenital malformation" admitted to one of four teaching hospital neonatal units between July 1988 and June 1990 with a birth weight of 1500 g or less or a gestational age less than 31 weeks were included.

Study size

The training group had 812 patients and the validation group 488.

Pretest probability

The overall rate of in-hospital mortality was 24.5%.

Type of validation

Grade II: The validation group was a separate sample from the same population, with data for the validation group gathered prospectively.

Comments

The clinical risk index for babies (CRIB) score is the easiest to use neonatal risk score. It was developed before surfactant was in widespread use, but a prospective evaluation in 720 patients (36% of whom received surfactant) showed that the variables in CRIB remained independent predictors of outcome. The authors caution appropriately that the CRIB score is most useful for comparing neonatal units and should not be used to determine the prognosis for individuals.

Reference

International Neonatal Network. The CRIB (clinical risk index for babies) score: a tool for assessing initial neonatal risk and comparing performance of neonatal intensive care units. Lancet 1993;342:193–198.

CLINICAL PREDICTION RULE

1. Add up the points below.

Risk factor	Score
Birth weight (g)	
1351–1500	0
851–1350	1
701–850	4
≤700	7
Gestational age (weeks)	
24–31	0
≤24	1
Congenital malformations	
None	0
Not acutely life-threatening	1
Acutely life-threatening	3
Maximum base excess during first 12 hours (mmol/L)	
≥7.0	0
−7.0 to −9.9	1
−10.0 to −14.9	2
≤−15.0	3
Minimum appropriate FiO_2 during first 12 hours	
≤0.40	0
0.41–0.60	2
0.61–0.90	3
0.91–1.00	4
Maximum appropriate FiO_2 during first 12 hours	
≤0.40	0
0.41–0.80	1
0.81–0.90	3
0.91–1.0	5
Total:	

2. The risk of in-hospital mortality and major cerebral abnormality for increasing CRIB scores is shown below.

CRIB score	In-hospital mortality	With major cerebral abnormality
0–5	7%	5%
6–10	37%	12%
11–15	68%	20%
>15	92%	20%

Neonatal Severity of Illness: Score for Neonatal Acute Physiology (SNAP)

Clinical question

What is the prognosis for infants in the neonatal intensive care unit (NICU)?

Population and setting

The scale was developed ad hoc by expert clinicians, who assigned points to varying degrees of physiologic derangement for 26 variables. The scale was validated on a group of consecutive admissions to the NICU. To be included, infants had to remain in the NICU at least 24 hours and have complete medical records. Late readmissions were not included.

Study size

A total of 1643 infants were studied.

Pretest probability

The mortality rate in the study group was 6.9%.

Type of validation

Grade II: The rule was developed ad hoc and validated in a group of patients at the author's institution.

Comments

This score is similar in design and conception to the Acute Physiology and Chronic Health Evaluation (APACHE) score for adults. It is a purely physiologic score, a strength because scores using diagnostic or therapeutic variables are more subject to local variation and are therefore less generalizable.

Reference

Richardson DK, Gray JE, McCormick MC, et al. Score for neonatal acute physiology: a physiologic severity index for neonatal intensive care. Pediatrics 1993;91:617–623.

CLINICAL PREDICTION RULE

1. Calculate the patient's SNAP score (usual range 0–42, theoretic range 0–127). For each variable, choose the worst measurement during the first 24 hours of admission. Note that you should use total or ionized calcium, not both.

Variable	1 Point	3 Points	5 Points	Your patient's points
MAP, maximum (mm Hg)[a]	66–80	81–100	>100	
MAP, minimum (mm Hg)[a]	30–35	20–29	<20	
Heart rate, maximum (beats/minute)	180–200	201–250	>250	
Heart rate, minimum (beats/minute)	80–90	40–79	<40	
Respiratory rate (breaths/minute)	60–100	>100		
Temperature (°F)	95–96	92–94.9	<92	
PaO_2 (mm Hg)	50–65	30–50	<30	
PaO_2/FiO_2 ratio (FiO_2 as a %)	2.5–3.5	0.30–2.49	<0.3	
$PaCO_2$ (mm Hg)	50–65	66–90	>90	
Oxygenation index[b]	0.07–0.20	0.21–0.40	>0.40	
Hematocrit, maximum (%)	66–70	>70		
Hematocrit, minimum (%)	30–35	20–29	<20	
White blood cell (WBC) count (cells/μl)	2000–5000	<2000		
Immature/total neutrophil ratio[c]	>0.21			
Absolute neutrophil count (% neutrophils × WBC)	500–999	<500		
Platelet count (cells/μl)	30,000–100,000	<30,000		
Blood urea nitrogen (mg/dl)	40–80	>80		
Serum creatinine (mg/dl)	1.2–2.4	2.5–4.0	>4.0	
Urine output (ml/kg/hr)	0.5–0.9	0.10–0.49	<0.1	
Indirect bilirubin				
Birth weight > 2 kg (mg/dl)	15–20	>20		
Birth weight ≤ 2 kg (mg/dl/kg)	5–10	>10		
Direct bilirubin (mg/dl)	≥2.0			
Sodium, maximum (mEq/l)	150–160	161–180	>180	
Sodium, minimum (mEq/l)	120–130	<120		
Potassium, maximum (mEq/l)	6.6–7.5	7.6–9.0	>9.0	
Potassium, minimum (mEq/l)	2.0–2.9	<2.0		
Total calcium, maximum (mg/dl)[d]	≥12			
Total calcium, minimum (mg/dl)[d]	5.0–6.9	<5.0		
Ionized calcium, maximum (mg/dl)[d]	≥1.4			
Ionized calcium, minimum (mg/dl)[d]	0.8–1.0	<0.8		
Glucose, maximum (mg/dl)	150–250	≥250		
Glucose, minimum (mg/dl)	30–40	<30		
Serum bicarbonate, maximum (mEq/l)	≥33			
Serum bicarbonate, minimum (mEq/l)	11–15	≤10		
Serum pH	7.20–7.30	7.10–7.19	<7.10	
Seizures	Single	Multiple		
Apnea	Responsive to stimulation	Unresponsive to stimulation	Complete apnea	
Stool guaiac	Positive			
			Total:	

[a]MAP = mean arterial pressure = ([systolic blood pressure] + [2 × (diastolic blood pressure)])/3.
[b]Oxygenation index = [(mean airway pressure) × (FiO_2) × 100]/PaO_2.
[c]Immature/total neutrophil ratio = (promyelocytes + myelocytes + metamyelocytes + bands-stabs)/total neutrophils.
[d]Use total or ionized calcium, not both.

2. Interpret the SNAP score using the table below.

Birth weight	SNAP score	No. of infants in this group	In-hospital mortality rate
300–749 g	0–9	3	33%
	10–19	24	42%
	>19	26	66%
750–999 g	0–9	13	0%
	10–19	66	20%
	>19	11	64%
1000–1499 g	0–9	76	0%
	10–19	113	6%
	>19	14	50%
>1500 g	0–9	853	0%
	10–19	369	4%
	>19	53	28%

Neonatal Severity of Illness: SNAP with Perinatal Extensions (SNAP-PE)

Clinical question

What is the prognosis for infants in the neonatal intensive care unit (NICU), taking into account both perinatal and physiologic variables?

Population and setting

The original SNAP score was developed ad hoc by expert clinicians, who assigned points to varying degrees of physiologic derangement for 26 variables. They then used a group of consecutive admissions to the NICU to test six SNAP-PE candidate models. Two-thirds of the patients were used to develop the six candidate models and one-third to test them. The best model was simplified and became the SNAP-PE.

Study size

Altogether, 1643 infants were studied.

Pretest probability

The mortality rate in the study group was 6.9%.

Type of validation

Grade II: The rule was developed ad hoc and validated in a group of patients at the author's institution.

Comments

This is an extension of the original SNAP score. The authors evaluated a number of possible extensions to the SNAP score and, using a training group/validation group approach, chose the best one. The data shown below are for all patients in the training and validation groups. The SNAP-PE has an area under the ROC curve of 0.93, excellent for this sort of model.

Reference

Richardson DK, Phibbs CS, Gray JE, et al. Birth weight and illness severity: independent predictors of neonatal mortality. Pediatrics 1993;91:969–975.

CLINICAL PREDICTION RULE

1. Calculate the patient's SNAP score (usual range 0–42, theoretic range 0–127). For each variable, choose the worst measurement during the first 24 hours of admission. Note that you should use total or ionized calcium, not both:

Variable	1 Point	3 Points	5 Points	Your patient's points
MAP, maximum (mm Hg)[a]	66–80	81–100	>100	
MAP, minimum (mm Hg)[a]	30–35	20–29	<20	
Heart rate, maximum (beats/minute)	180–200	201–250	>250	
Heart rate, minimum (beats/minute)	80–90	40–79	<40	
Respiratory rate (breaths/minute)	60–100	>100		
Temperature (°F)	95–96	92.0–94.9	<92	
PaO_2 (mm Hg)	50–65	30–50	<30	
PaO_2/FiO_2 ratio (FiO_2 as a %)	2.5–3.5	0.30–2.49	<0.3	
$PaCO_2$ (mm Hg)	50–65	66–90	>90	
Oxygenation index[b]	0.07–0.20	0.21–0.40	>0.40	
Hematocrit, maximum (%)	66–70	>70		
Hematocrit, minimum (%)	30–35	20–29	<20	
White blood cell (WBC) count (cells/μl)	2000–5000	<2000		
Immature/total neutrophil ratio[c]	>0.21			
Absolute neutrophil count (% neutrophils × WBC)	500–999	<500		
Platelet count (cells/μl)	30,000–100,000	<30,000		
Blood urea nitrogen (mg/dl)	40–80	>80		
Serum creatinine (mg/dl)	1.2–2.4	2.5–4.0	>4.0	
Urine output (ml/kg/hr)	0.5–0.9	0.10–0.49	<0.1	
Indirect bilirubin				
Birthweight > 2 kg (mg/dl)	15–20	>20		
Birthweight ≤ 2 kg (mg/dl/kg)	5–10	>10		
Direct bilirubin (mg/dl)	≥2.0			
Sodium, maximum (mEq/l)	150–160	161–180	>180	
Sodium, minimum (mEq/l)	120–130	<120		
Potassium, maximum (mEq/l)	6.6–7.5	7.6–9.0	>9.0	
Potassium, minimum (mEq/l)	2.0–2.9	<2.0		
Total calcium, maximum (mg/dl)[d]	≥12			
Total calcium, minimum (mg/dl)[d]	5.0–6.9	<5.0		
Ionized calcium, maximum (mg/dl)[d]	≥1.4			
Ionized calcium, minimum (mg/dl)[d]	0.8–1.0	< 0.8		
Glucose, maximum (mg/dl)	150–250	≥ 250		
Glucose, minimum (mg/dl)	30–40	<30		
Serum bicarbonate, maximum (mEq/L)	≥33			
Serum bicarbonate, minimum (mEq/L)	11–15	≤10		
Serum pH	7.20–7.30	7.10–7.19	<7.10	
Seizures	Single	Multiple		
Apnea	Responsive to stimulation	Unresponsive to stimulation	Complete apnea	
Stool guaiac	Positive			
			Total:	

[a]MAP = mean arterial pressure = ([systolic blood pressure] + [2 × (diastolic blood pressure)])/3.
[b]Oxygenation index = [(mean airway pressure) × (F/O_2) × 100)/PaO_2].
[c]Immature/total neutrophil ratio = (promyelocytes + myelocytes + metamyelocytes + bands-stabs)/total neutrophils.
[d]Use total or ionized calcium, not both.

2. Use the SNAP score from above to calculate the SNAP-PE score.

Item	Points
Enter the SNAP score from the first 24 hours of NICU admission at right:	____
Add points for each of the following characteristics if present:	
Birth weight ≤749 g	+30
Birth weight 750–999 g	+10
Apgar <7 at 5 minutes	+10
Small for gestational age (<5th percentile)	+5
Total SNAP-PE score:	

3. Interpret the SNAP-PE score below.

	<1500 g		≥1500 g	
SNAP-PE score	No. in this group	Mortality	No. in this group	Mortality
0–9	52	0%	768	0%
10–19	108	0.9%	367	1.3%
20–29	87	14.0%	102	11.0%
30–39	34	38.0%	31	32.0%
40–69	57	53.0%	7	57.0%
≥70	8	75.0%	—	—

CRITICAL CARE

Pediatric Risk of Mortality (PRISM) for Pediatric Intensive Care

Clinical question

What is the risk of death among children in the pediatric intensive care unit (ICU)?

Population and setting

The population used to validate the rule was a group of 270 children admitted consecutively to the pediatric ICU at the Royal Hospital of Sick Children in Glasgow, Scotland. The median age was 19 months (range 3 days to 18.6 years); 157 of 270 were boys; 146 of 270 were admitted postoperatively; and the median length of stay in the ICU was 2 days. For validation of the pre-ICU PRISM score, patients came from four tertiary care medical centers in the United States. All patients in the latter study were emergency admissions to the pediatric ICU; neonatal admissions were excluded.

Study size

The validation set had 270 patients in the Scottish study and 390 in the pre-ICU American study.

Pretest probability

Of the 270 children, 29 (10.7%) did not survive in the Scottish study; mortality was approximately 15% in the American study.

Type of validation

Scottish study: Grade I: The validation group was from a distinct population. The rule was developed in one group of patients and validated in a separate group.
American study: Grade II: The test set was a separate sample from the same population, with data for the test set gathered prospectively.

Comments

This prospective validation showed that the PRISM score, developed in the United States, performed just as well in an independent population of Scottish children. The sensitivity in postoperative patients (17%) was much lower than that for nonoperative patients (71%), although the specificity was similar for both groups (100% vs. 96%). This was largely because the PRISM score failed to identify 10 of 11 postoperative cardiac deaths. The American study uses scores calculated just prior to admission to the pediatric ICU.

References

Balakrishnan G, Aitchison T, Hallworth D, Morton NS. Prospective evaluation of the Pediatric Risk of Mortality (PRISM) score. Arch Dis Child 1992;67:196–200.

Pollack M, Ruttimann UE, Getson PR. Pediatric Risk of Mortality (PRISM) score. Crit Care Med 1988;16:1110–1116.

CLINICAL PREDICTION RULE

1. Calculate the PRISM physiology score for your pediatric patient during the first day of admission (range 0 to 76 points):

Variable/age	Range	Points
Systolic blood pressure (mmHg)		
0–1 Year	130–160	2
	55–65	2
	>160	6
	40–54	6
	<40	7
>1 Year	150–200	2
	65–75	2
	>200	6
	50–64	6
	<50	7
Diastolic blood pressure (mmHg)		
All ages	>110	6
Heart rate (beats/minute)		
0–1 Year	<90 or >160	4
>1 Year	<80 or >150	4
Respiratory rate (breaths/min)		
0–1 Year	61–90	1
	>90 or apnea	5
>1 Year	51–70	1
	>70 or apnea	5
PaO_2/FiO_2 ratio		
All ages	200–300	2
	<200	3
$PaCO_2$ (mmHg)		
All ages	51–65	1
	>65	5
Glasgow Coma Score		
All ages	<8	6
Pupillary reaction		
All ages	Unequal or dilated	4
	Fixed and dilated	10
PT/PTT ratio		
All ages	1.5 Times control	2
Total bilirubin (mg/dl)		
>1 Month	>3.5	6
Potassium (mEq/l)		
All ages	3.0–3.5	1
	6.5–7.5	1
	<3.0 or >7.5	5
Calcium (mg/dl)		
All ages	7.0–8.0	2
	12.0–15.0	2
	<7.0 or >15.0	6
Glucose (mg/dl)		
All ages	40–60	4
	250–400	4
	<40 or >400	8
Bicarbonate (mEq/L)		
All ages	<16 or >32	3
	Total PRISM physiology score:	

PT/PTT = prothrombin time/partial thromboplastin time.

2. Use the PRISM physiology score, the age in months, and the operative status (1 if postoperative, 0 if nonoperative) to estimate the risk of death during this admission to the pediatric ICU.

$$\text{Score} = [0.207 \times (\text{PRISM score})] - [0.005 \times (\text{age in months})] - [0.433 \times (\text{operative status})] - 4.782$$

$$\text{Probability of ICU death} = e^{\text{score}}/(1 + e^{\text{score}})$$

3. The pre-ICU PRISM scores were calculated in a prospective, independent validation in four U.S. tertiary care hospitals. The risk of mortality is given by these equations.

$$\text{Score} = [0.197 \times (\text{PRISM score})] - 4.705$$

$$\text{Probability of ICU death} = e^{\text{score}}/(1 + e^{\text{score}})$$

14

Pulmonary Disease

PNEUMONIA AND COUGH

Diagnosis of *Pneumocystis* Pneumonia in Outpatients

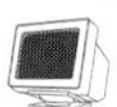

Clinical question

Which ambulatory patients with risk factors for human immunodeficiency virus (HIV) disease and respiratory symptoms have *Pneumocystis carinii* pneumonia (PCP)?

Population and setting

Consecutive patients with HIV risk factors and respiratory symptoms presenting to an urgent care center in San Francisco were included. Most (88%) were male; 76% were gay or bisexual; 20% were intravenous drug users; and 8% had a sexual partner in a risk group.

Study size

Although 279 patients were studied, only 125 were used in the logistic regression owing to missing data.

Pretest probability

Altogether, 24.8% of patients had *Pneumocystis carinii* pneumonia.

Type of validation

Grade IV: The training group was used as the validation group.

Comments

Given the absence of prospective validation, this rule is appropriate to identify patients at high risk but should not be used to rule out PCP.

Reference

Katz MH, Baron RB, Grady D. Risk stratification of ambulatory patients suspected of Pneumocystis pneumonia. Arch Intern Med 1991;151:105–110.

CLINICAL PREDICTION RULE

1. Determine whether the patient has diffuse perihilar infiltrates and the number of the following abnormal findings.

Mouth lesions
Presence of a lactate dehydrogenase (LDH) level > 220 U/L
Erythrocyte sedimentation rate (ESR) of 50 mm/hr or more

2. Identify the patient's risk group based on these characteristics.

Risk group	Characteristics	No. with PCP/ no. in group	LR for PCP
High	Diffuse perihilar infiltrates	21/25 (84%)	15.9
High–intermediate	No diffuse perihilar infiltrates and two or three abnormal findings	7/15 (47%)	2.7
Low–intermediate	No diffuse perihilar infiltrates and one abnormal finding	3/35 (9%)	0.3
Low	No diffuse perihilar infiltrates and no abnormal findings	0/50	0.1

LR = likelihood ratio.

Likelihood of Pneumonia in Patients with Cough

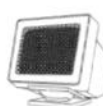

Clinical question

Which outpatients with acute cough have pneumonia on radiography?

Population and setting

All nonpregnant adults seeking medical care for the first time for coughs of less than 1 month duration at an Army Medical Center emergency department were included. Patients were excluded if they had a heart rate $>$ 160 beats per minute, temperature $>$ 104°F, systolic blood pressure $<$ 90 mm Hg, or if they arrived by ambulance. Only 25% declined to participate. The mean age was 40 years; 51% were female.

Study size

A total of 483 patients were studied, plus another 1305 to calculate the specificity.

Pretest probability

Of these patients, 2.6% had pneumonia on radiography and another 2.6% had "a possible infiltrate and equivocal pneumonia."

Type of validation

Grade III: The validation group was a separate sample from the same population, although data for both training and validation groups were gathered at the same time. A jackknife validation method was used, increasing the accuracy of this approach to validation.

Comments

The major limitation of this study is that there was no clear set of criteria for interpreting the radiographs. Otherwise, it is a useful rule and is well validated.

Reference

Diehr P, Wood RW, Bushyhead J, et al. Prediction of pneumonia in outpatients with acute cough: a statistical approach. *J Chronic Dis* 1984;37:215–225.

CLINICAL PREDICTION RULE

1. Add up the number of points for your patient.

Finding	Points
Rhinorrhea	−2
Sore throat	−1
Night sweats	1
Myalgia	1
Sputum all day	1
Respiratory rate > 25	2
Temperature ≥ 100°F	2
Total:	

2. Based on the number of points, find the percent with pneumonia.

Score	No. with score	With pneumonia
−3	140	0%
−2	556	0.7%
−1	512	1.6%
0	323	2.2%
1	136	8.8%
2	58	10.3%
3	16	25.0%
≥4	11	29.4%

Pneumonia Prognosis Index

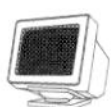

Clinical question

What is the prognosis for patients with community-acquired pneumonia?

Population and setting

The original study by Fine et al. included adults with symptoms and radiographic evidence of pneumonia; they were excluded if it was a readmission or they were HIV-positive. The second validation in nursing home patients by Mylotte and colleagues included 100 patients admitted from a nursing home to the hospital and 58 patients managed in the nursing home without hospital admission. The validation by Flanders et al. used 1024 randomly selected patients in 22 community hospitals.

Study size

Fine et al. developed the rule from an administrative data set with 14,199 patients and validated it in a second group of 2287 community-based and nursing home patients. Mylotte et al. validated it in 158 nursing home patients.

Pretest probability

Risk of death in the original study by Fine et al. was 5.2%; and in Mylotte et al.'s nursing home study it was 22.1%.

Type of validation

Grade I: The validation group was from a distinct population. The rule was developed in one group of patients and validated in another.

Comments

The original study by Fine et al. included a broad spectrum of community and nursing patients. A second independent validation of the rule was in a population of patients who were admitted from a nursing home or treated in a nursing home. A subsequent prospective validation in a community setting is also reported and shows that the rule discriminates well.

References

Fine MJ, Auble TE, Yealy DM, et al. A prediction rule to identify low-risk patients with community-acquired pneumonia. N Engl J Med 1997;336:243–250.

Flanders WD, Tucker G, Krishnadasan A, et al. Validation of the Pneumonia Severity Index: importance of study-specific recalibration. J Gen Intern Med 1999;14:333–340.

Mylotte JM, Naughton B, Saludades C, Maszarovics Z. Validation and application of the Pneumonia Prognosis Index to nursing home residents with pneumonia. J Am Geriatr Soc 1998;46:1538–1544.

CLINICAL PREDICTION RULE

1. Count up the number of points for your patient.

Risk factor	Points
Enter the age in years at right	
If female, subtract 10 points	−10
Nursing home resident	10
Co-morbidities	
Neoplasm	30
Liver disease	20
Heart failure	10
Stroke	10
Renal	10
Physical examination findings	
Altered mental status	20
Respiratory rate ≥ 30/min	20
Systolic BP < 90 mmHg	20
Temp < 35°C or ≥40°C	15
Pulse ≥ 125/min	10
Laboratory and radiographic findings	
Arterial pH < 7.35	30
BUN ≥ 30 mg/dl	20
Sodium < 130 mmol/L	20
Glucose ≥ 250 mg/dl	10
Hct < 30%	10
PO_2 < 50 mmHg	10
Pleural effusion	10
Total:	

2. Determine your patient's risk class.

Characteristic	Risk class
Under age 50 and no co-morbidities, abnormal physical examination findings, or laboratory or radiographic findings from the list above	I
Not class I (above) but:	
<70 points	II
71–90 Points	III
91–130 Points	IV
>130 Points	V

3. The risk of death and length of stay (where data are available) are shown below.

	Original validation cohort (community-based and nursing home) of Fine et al.			
Risk class	No. of inpatients	Inpatient mortality	Length of stay (days)	Outpatient mortality
I	772	0.1%	5	0.5%
II	477	0.9%	6	0.4%
III	326	1.2%	7	0.0%
IV	486	9.0%	9	12.5%
V	226	27.1%	11	12.5%

Note: The numbers are too small to be meaningful for risk class I and II in nursing home patients. Patients were not randomized to inpatient or outpatient treatment in

Fine et al.'s study, so one can assume that selection bias for managing healthier patients in the outpatient setting occurred.

Fine et al. recommended that patients in risk class I or II be considered for outpatient therapy and those in risk class IV and V definitely be hospitalized. Of course, the final decision on the type of therapy requires consideration of all relevant patient factors.

4. Results from two prospective validations.

	Community hospitals Flanders et al.)		Nursing home (Mylotte et al.)	
Risk class	No.	Mortality	No.	Mortality
I	14	0%	—	—
II	123	0%	—	—
III	585	1.8%	21	4.8%
IV	290	13.1%	50	12.0%
V	12	0%	85	32.9%

Prognosis in Community-Acquired Pneumonia (Geriatric)

Clinical question

What is the prognosis for community-acquired pneumonia in the elderly?

Population and setting

Patients over age 65 with an initial working diagnosis of pneumonia assigned by their admitting physician and a chest radiograph during the first 48 hours that was consistent with pneumonia were included. The following patients were excluded: those with HIV disease, previous organ transplant, receiving chemotherapy within the past 2 months, transfer from another hospital, readmission within 10 days from a prior acute care hospitalization, or discharge or death on the day of admission. Variables used to develop the rule were recorded within 24 hours of admission. This project was done as part of the Pneumonia Module of the Medicare Quality Indicator System.

Study size

The training group had 1000 patients and consisted of a random sample of patients from four states (Massachusetts, Maryland, New Hampshire, West Virginia). The validation group had 1356 patients and was a random sample of similar patients from each state in the United States. The validation group had more males (51% vs. 45%), fewer white patients (88% vs. 91%), and more patients from a skilled nursing facility (30% vs. 24%) than the training group.

Pretest probability

In the validation group, 12% of patients died, 33% went to a skilled nursing facility, 61% went home, and the rest went elsewhere.

Type of validation

Grade III: The rule was developed using one group of patients and then was validated in another group of similar patients.

Comments

This rule was developed and validated using a retrospective chart audit. Because prospective data collection can sometimes give different results, it should be prospectively validated before being applied.

Reference

Conte HA, Chen Y-T, Mehal W, et al. A prognostic rule for elderly patients admitted with community-acquired pneumonia. Am J Med 1999;106:20–28.

CLINICAL PREDICTION RULE

1. Determine your patient's risk score.

Predictor	Points
Age ≥ 85 years	1
Presence of co-morbid condition[a]	2
Impaired motor response[b]	1
Abnormal vital signs (temp > 36.1°C, SBP < 90 mm Hg or heart rate > 110 beats/min)	2
Serum creatinine level ≥ 1.5 mg/dl	1
Total:	

SBP = systolic blood pressure

[a]Co-morbid conditions include acute or chronic leukemia, Hodgkin's or non-Hodgkin's lymphoma, multiple myeloma, any cancer with local or distant metastases, hepatic failure, cirrhosis, chemotherapy or radiotherapy within the last year (but not 2 months before admission), or a collagen vascular disease.

[b]Impaired motor response is defined as failure to exhibit a motor response to verbal stimuli (localization of painful stimuli alone, flexion withdrawal, decorticate/decerebrate posturing, or no response).

2. Determine the risk of in-hospital mortality.

Risk score	In-hospital mortality
0	4%
1–2	11%
3–4	23%
>4	41%

Evaluation of Chronic Cough

Clinical question

What are the most likely diagnoses among patients presenting with chronic cough?

Population and setting

In the Mello et al. study, consecutive immune-competent outpatients referred for evaluation of chronic cough to a pulmonology clinic were included. The cough was of at least 3 weeks' duration. The mean age was 53 years (range 15–83 years); 73% were female. In the Marchesani et al. study, patients were included if they had been referred for evaluation of cough of at least 4 weeks' duration, no obvious cause was found, and it did not respond to initial treatment by their physician.

Study size

A total of 88 patients were studied by Mello et al.

Pretest probability

This parameter is not applicable.

Type of validation

Mello et al.: Grade IV: The training group was used as the validation group.
Marchesani et al.: Grade I: The test set was from a distinct population. The rule was developed in one group of patients and validated in another.

Comments

This simple rule is informative rather than predictive, as it helps guide the evaluation of patients with chronic cough but does not help make a specific diagnosis. The systematic evaluation in both studies included chest and sinus radiography, spirometry with methacholine challenge, skin testing, and occasionally esophagogastroduodenectomy or pH monitoring.

References

Marchesani F, Cecarini L, Pela R, Sanguinetti CM. Causes of chronic persistent cough in adult patients: the results of a systematic management protocol. Monaldi Arch Chest Dis 1998;53:510–514.

Mello CJ, Irwin RS, Curley FJ. Predictive values of the character, timing, and complications of chronic cough in diagnosis its cause. Arch Intern Med 1996;156:997–1003.

CLINICAL PREDICTION RULE

Unexplained chronic cough is generally caused by gastroesophageal reflux disease (GERD), postnasal drip syndrome (PND), or asthma.

Mello study
Among patients with the following three characteristics, 99.4% had either GERD, PND, or asthma as the cause of their chronic cough.

Nonsmoker
Not receiving an angiotensin-converting enzyme (ACE) inhibitor drug
Normal or nearly normal and stable chest radiograph

Marchesani study
Among patients with cough for at least 4 weeks, no obvious cause, and lack of response to "conventional therapy prescribed by general practitioners":

56% had PND, usually caused by sinusitis
14% had asthma
5% had GERD
6% had PND and GERD
1% had asthma and GERD
18% had chronic bronchitis

Likelihood of Pulmonary Infiltrates in Patients with Fever or Respiratory Symptoms

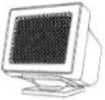

Clinical question

Which patients presenting with fever or respiratory symptoms have pulmonary infiltrates seen by chest radiography?

Population and setting

Consecutive patients more than 15 years old presenting with fever or respiratory symptoms to an emergency department who underwent radiography were included. The mean age was 43 years; 46% were male.

Study size

The training group had 1134 patients and the validation group 302.

Pretest probability

In the validation group, 25.8% had pneumonia, as did 12.4% in the training group.

Type of validation

Grade I: The validation group was from a distinct population. The rule was developed in one group of patients and validated in another.

Comments

This is an excellent clinical rule—easy to use and well validated. It was validated again in a study by Emerman et al., where it was found to be somewhat less sensitive than the judgment of experienced physicians (71% vs. 86%) but more specific (67% vs. 58%) and overall more accurate (68% vs. 60%).

References

Emerman CL, Dawson N, Speroff T, et al. Comparison of physician judgment and decision aids for ordering chest radiographs for pneumonia in outpatients. Ann Emerg Med 1991;20:1215–1219.

Heckerling PS, Tape TG, Wigton RS, et al. Clinical prediction rule for pulmonary infiltrates. Ann Intern Med 1990;113:664–670.

CLINICAL PREDICTION RULE

1. Count the number of points for your patient (range 0–5).

Finding	Points
Temperature > 38.7°C	1
Pulse > 100 beats/minute	1
Rales	1
Decreased breath sounds	1
Absence of asthma	1
Total:	

2. Add up the number of points and use the table below to interpret the results. Note that two sets of pretest probability are given, 28% and 19%.

	% With infiltrate	
Points	(28% Pretest probability)	(19% Pretest probability)
0	3%	1.6%
1	9%	5%
2	24%	14%
3	51%	35%
4	77%	63%
5	91%	85%

Prognosis with Pneumonia and Acute Respiratory Failure

Clinical question

Which critically ill patients admitted to the intensive care unit (ICU) with acute bacterial pneumonia and acute respiratory failure will survive?

Population and setting

All adult patients admitted to the ICU of a French hospital with acute bacterial pneumonia (confirmed by clinical and radiologic data) and acute respiratory failure (not defined) were included. The mean age was 52 years (range 18–86 years); 80% were male; most (70%) were on artificial ventilation.

Study size

There were 96 patients in the validation group.

Pretest probability

In-hospital mortality rate was 57%.

Type of validation

Grade I: The validation group was from a distinct population. The rule was developed in one group of patients and validated in another.

Comments

Generalizability may be an issue, as French hospitals use different criteria for admission to their small ICUs than American hospitals. This rule uses the Simplified Acute Physiology Score, developed originally to assist in ICU prognostication.

Reference

Durocher A, Saulnier F, Beuscart, et al. A comparison of three severity score indexes in an evaluation of serious bacterial pneumonia. Intensive Care Med 1988;14:39–43.

CLINICAL PREDICTION RULE

1. Calculate the Simplified Acute Physiology Score for your patient:

	Points									
Variable	4	3	2	1	0	1	2	3	4	Total
Age (years)					≤40	41–55	56–65	66–75	>75	
Heart rate	≥180	140–179	110–139		70–109		55–69	40–54	<40	
SBP (mm Hg)	≥190		150–189		80–149		55–79		<55	
Body temp. (°C)	≥41	39.0–40.9		38.5–38.9	36.0–37.4	34.0–35.9	32.0–33.9	30.0–31.9	<30.0	
Spontaneous respiration rate	≥50	35–49		25–34	12–24	10–11	6–9		<6	
or ventilation on CPAP								Yes		
Urinary output (L/24hr)			≥5.0	3.5–4.99	0.7–3.49		0.50–0.69	0.20–0.49	<0.2	
Blood urea (mmol/L)	≥55.0	36.0–54.9	29.0–35.9	7.5–26.9	3.5–7.4	3.5				
Hematocrit (%)	≥60.0		50.0–59.9	46.0–49.9	30.0–45.9		20.0–29.9		<20.0	
WBC count ($10^3/mm^3$)	≥40.0		20.0–39.9	15.0–19.9	3.0–14.9		1.0–2.9		<1.0	
Serum glucose (mmol/L)	≥44.5	27.8–44.4		14.0–27.7	3.9–13.9		2.8–3.8	1.6–2.7	<1.6	
Serum potassium (mEq/L)	≥7.0	6.0–6.9		5.5–5.9	3.5–5.4	3.0–3.4	2.5–2.9		<2.5	
Serum sodium (mEq/L)	≥180	161–179	156–160	151–155	130–150		120–129	110–119	<110	
Serum HCO_3 (mEq/L)		≥40.0		30.0–39.9	20.0–29.9	10.0–19.9		5.0–9.9	<5.0	
GCS					13–15	10–12	7–9	4–6	3	
								Total:		

SBP = systolic blood pressure; CPAP = continuous positive airway pressure; WBC = white blood cells; GCS = Glasgow Coma Scale.

2. The following mortality rates were found.

Score	Mortality rate
≥17	83.3% (n = 30)
13–16	55.3% (n = 38)
≤12	32.1% (n = 28)

Risk of Nosocomial Pneumonia in the Intensive Care Unit

Clinical question

Which patients in the intensive care unit (ICU) for at least 72 hours will develop nosocomial pneumonia?

Population and setting

Consecutive adult patients admitted to the ICU of a university hospital and staying at least 72 hours were included. The mean age was 57 years; 57% were male.

Study size

Altogether, 203 patients were studied.

Pretest probability

Of these patients, 12.8% developed a nosocomial pneumonia.

Type of validation

Grade IV: The training group was used as the validation group.

Comments

The terms "rapidly fatal" and "ultimately fatal" disease are not clearly defined. Furthermore, the rule has not been prospectively validated. This rule should therefore be used with caution.

Reference

Joshi N, Localio AR, Hamory BH. A predictive risk index for nosocomial pneumonia in the intensive care unit. Am J Med 1992;93:135–142.

CLINICAL PREDICTION RULE

1. Identify which risk factors your patient has and multiply these scores.

Risk factor	Score if risk factor is present
Age > 60 years	2.0
Ultimately fatal disease	3.0
Rapidly fatal disease	4.0
Upper abdominal/thoracic surgery	4.0
Intubation	2.0
Altered consciousness	1.5
Nasogastric tube	6.5
H_2-blocker therapy	2.0
Recent bronchoscopy	3.0
Product:	

2. The probability of pneumonia can be found in the table below.

Product	Probability of pneumonia
0	0%
3	1%
5	1%
8	2%
10	3%
12	3%
15	4%
20	5%
30	8%
40	11%
50	14%
60	18%
70	21%
80	25%
100	33%
120	43%
140	54%
160	67%
180	82%
200	100%

3. To calculate an exact estimate, multiply the "Product" from the table by 0.0025. This is the odds of pneumonia.

4. A patient is considered high risk if the odds are >0.11 (sensitivity 85%, specificity 66% for nosocomial pneumonia).

5. If desired, convert the odds to probability.

$$\text{Probability of nosocomial pneumonia} = \frac{\text{odds}}{(1 - \text{odds})}$$

This rule had an area under the ROC curve of 0.86, with a 27% positive predictive value and a 97% negative predictive value. That means that 97% of patients considered at low risk did not develop a nosocomial pneumonia, and 27% of the high risk patients did develop pneumonia.

Example: a patient with rapidly fatal disease, upper abdominal/thoracic surgery, and nasogastric tube has a product of $4 \times 4 \times 6.5 = 104$. Multiply this product by 0.0025 to get the odds of 0.26. Convert them to a probability: $0.26/(1 - 0.26) = 35\%$.

ACUTE RESPIRATORY DISTRESS SYNDROME

Prognosis for Acute Respiratory Distress Syndrome

Clinical question

Which patients with acute respiratory distress syndrome (ARDS) will have a complicated course (early death or prolonged intubation)?

Population and setting

Adult patients at a tertiary medical center with ARDS diagnosed by standard criteria were included. Patients had to have all of the following: (1) acute respiratory failure requiring intubation; (2) rapid development of diffuse bilateral infiltrates; (3) recent exposure to an agent known to precipitate acute long injury; (4) pulmonary occlusion pressure < 18 mm Hg or absence of echocardiographic evidence of cardiogenic pulmonary edema; (5) total respiratory system compliance ≤ 50 ml/cm H_2O; and (6) severe hypoxemia.

Study size

Altogether, 126 patients were used to develop the rule and 50 patients to validate it prospectively.

Pretest probability

At day four, 72% were defined as having a complicated course. At day seven, 75% had a complicated course. Mortality for patients with a complicated course was 64% at seven days.

Type of validation

Grade II: The test set was a separate sample from the same population, with data for the test set gathered prospectively.

Comments

The radiograph viewers and researchers gathering clinical data did not participate in the care of the study patients. This is a well validated rule. The major limitation is the small size of the validation set, but this is understandable given the relative rarity of the condition.

Reference

Heffner JE, Brown LK, Barbieri CA, et al. Prospective validation of an acute respiratory distress syndrome predictive score. Am J Respir Crit Care Med 1995;152: 1518–1526.

CLINICAL PREDICTION RULE

1. Calculate the ARDS risk score.

Variable	Points
Chest radiograph compared with day 0	
Normalization of the radiograph	0
Clinically important radiographic improvement	1
Relative stability of radiographic infiltrates	2
Clinically important radiographic worsening	4
PaO_2/PAO_2 (ratio of arterial/alveolar oxygen tension)	
≥ 0.8	0
≥ 0.06 and <0.8	1
≥ 0.4 and <0.6	2
≥ 0.2 and <0.4	3
<0.2	4
Applied positive end-expiratory pressure (PEEP) (cm H_2O)	
0–5	0
6–8	1
9–11	2
12–14	3
≥ 15	4
Total:	

2. Interpret the risk score. A patient with a score ≥ 2.5 is considered at "high risk." Outcomes for 50 low risk and high risk patients in the validation study are shown below.

	Day 4 (50 total patients)		Day 7 (44 total patients left)	
Risk group	Complicated course ($n = 36$)	Death ($n = 24$)	Complicated course ($n = 33$)	Death ($n = 21$)
Low	16%	10%	23%	16%
High	56%	38%	52%	32%

OBSTRUCTIVE SLEEP APNEA

Diagnosis of Sleep Apnea Syndrome

Clinical question

Which patients referred for sleep studies actually have sleep apnea syndrome?

Population studied

Consecutive patients referred for a sleep study to a sleep clinic, which is the sole referral center for the province of Alberta, were included. A total of 83 of 263 (31.5%) did not participate owing to patient refusal ($n = 34$), a severe cardiac, neurologic, or pulmonary condition ($n = 23$), previous sleep apnea diagnosis ($n = 7$), use of tranquilizers or antidepressants ($n = 8$), or other reasons ($n = 11$). The mean age was 46 years; 75% were male.

Study size

Altogether, 180 patients were studied.

Pretest probability

Of these patients, 45% had sleep apnea syndrome.

Type of validation

Grade IV: The training group was used as the validation group.

Comments

The strength of this study is the complete capture of a referral population, making it more generalizable. The weakness is the lack of prospective validation and some potential for misinterpretation of predictor variables ("habitual snorer" and "history of gasping from partner"). It should be used with caution.

Reference

Flemons WW, Whitelow WA, Brant R, Remmers JE. Likelihood ratios for a sleep apnea clinical prediction rule. Am J Respir Crit Care Med 1994;150:1279–1285.

CLINICAL PREDICTION RULE

1. Count how many of the following historical features your patient has.

Habitual snoring
Partner reports nocturnal choking/gasping

2. Find the row with your patient's neck circumference, then go to the column that reflects the hypertensive status and the number of historical features present.

	Score, by number of historical features					
	Not hypertensive			Hypertensive		
Neck circumference (cm)	None	One	Both	None	One	Both
28	0	0	1	0	1	2
30	0	0	1	1	2	4
32	0	1	2	1	3	5
34	1	2	3	2	4	8
36	1	3	5	4	6	11
38	2	4	7	5	9	16
40	3	6	10	8	13	22
42	5	8	14	11	18	30
44	7	12	20	15	25	42
46	10	16	28	21	35	58
48	14	23	38	29	48	80
50	19	32	53	40	66	110

3. Finally, interpret the number of points from the above table as follows (an apnea-hypopnea index > 10 is diagnostic of sleep apnea syndrome).

Sleep apnea clinical score	Likelihood ratio	Probability of sleep apnea syndrome (based on pretest probability of 45%)
≤5	0.25 (0.15–0.42)[a]	17%
5.01–10.0	1.09 (0.62–1.92)	47%
10.01–15	2.03 (0.94–4.38)	62%
>15	5.17 (2.54–10.51)	81%

[a]Numbers in parentheses are the 95% confidence interval.

ASTHMA AND CHRONIC OBSTRUCTIVE PULMONARY DISEASE

Asthma in Adults

Clinical question

Which adult patients with asthma are likely to require hospitalization during the next year?

Population and setting

Patients age 18–50 years with moderate to severe asthma, on daily therapy for asthma, and with at least three visits to their physician during the previous year were included. The mean age was 38.4 years; 67% were female; and 36% were members of an ethnic minority (Hispanic, Asian, African American, or Native American).

Study size

A total of 323 patients were studied.

Pretest probability

Of these patients, 5.8% were hospitalized during the 1-year follow-up.

Type of validation

Grade IV: The training group was used as the validation group.

Comments

This rule can help identify outpatients at higher than average risk for asthma complications and who might benefit from more intensive educational efforts. It should be used with caution, as it has not been prospectively validated.

Reference

Dominic L, German D, Lulla S, Thomas RG, Wilson SR. Prospective study of hospitalization for asthma. Am J Respir Crit Care 1995;151:647–655.

CLINICAL PREDICTION RULE

Upper number is total children in group; lower number is children requiring hospitalization.

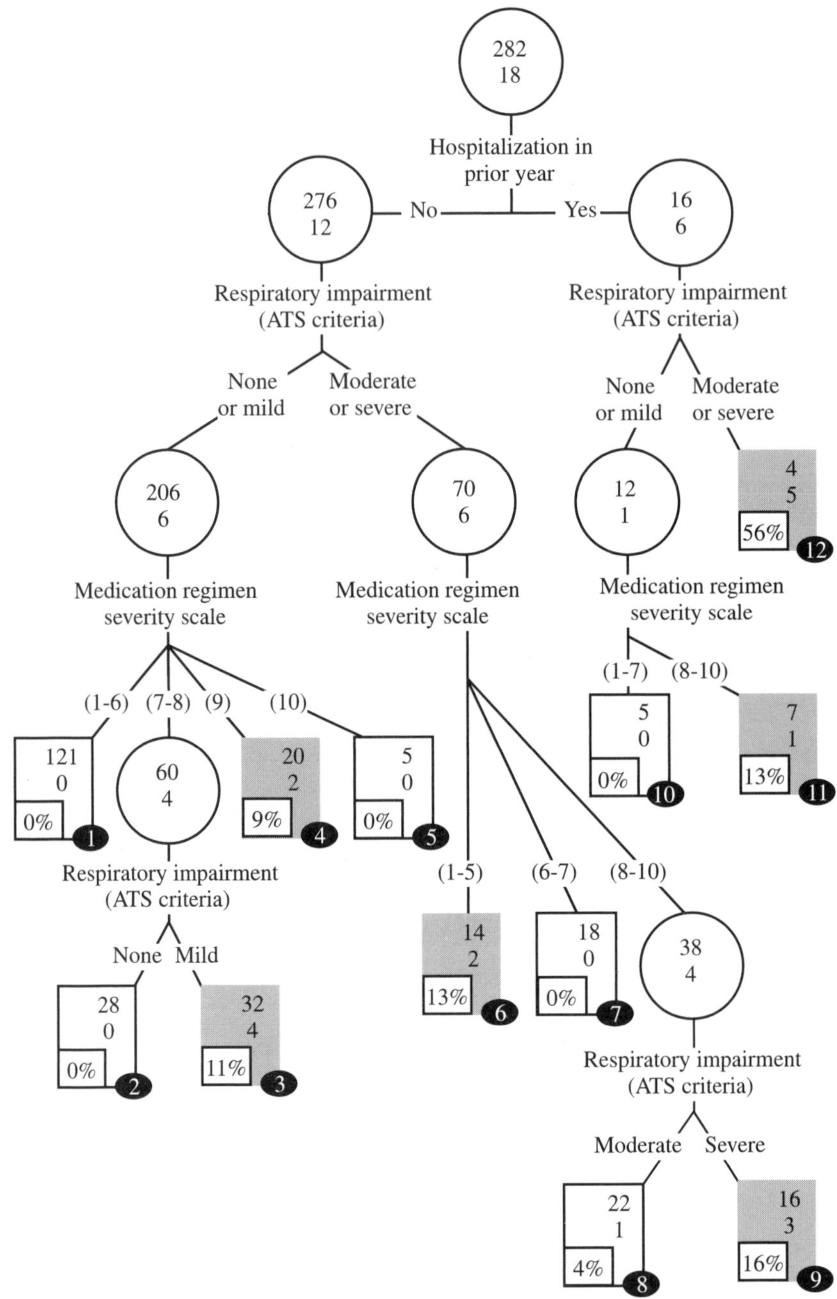

CYSTIC FIBROSIS

Survival with Cystic Fibrosis

Clinical question

What is the prognosis for patients with cystic fibrosis?

Population and setting

Patients referred to a British hospital with a diagnosis of cystic fibrosis were included. The rule was developed in patients seen between 1979 and 1987 and followed until 1989 or death. It was validated in a prospective cohort recruited between 1988 and 1993 and followed for 1 year or until their death. The age range in the validation group was 13–45 years; half were male.

Study size

The training group had 403 patients and the validation group 100.

Pretest probability

Of the study patients, 50.4% died during the study period.

Type of validation

Grade II: The validation group was a separate sample from the same population, with data for the validation group gathered prospectively.

Comments

Because this score was developed using data from the 1970s and 1980s and validated during the 1990s, it may underestimate survival today. For example, quinolones were not widely used until the 1990s. Note that the outcomes are approximations only and were extrapolated from a survival graph in the original article.

Reference

Hayllar K, Williams SG, Wise AE, et al. A prognostic model for the prediction of survival in cystic fibrosis. Thorax 1997;52:313–317.

CLINICAL PREDICTION RULE

1. Calculate the predictive index.

Variable	Points
Hepatomegaly present	0.99
Height (meters)	+ height × 1.54
% FEV1 of predicted	− % × 0.59
% FVC of predicted	− % × 0.038
WBC (10^9 cells/L)	+ WBC × 0.09
Total:	

FEV1 = forced expiratory volume in 1 second; FVC = forced vital capacity; WBC = white blood cells.

Example: a patient with a height of 1.54 meters, hepatomegaly, FVC = 50% predicted, FEV1 = 35% predicted, and WBC = 20 × 10^9 cells/L has the following predictive index (PI).

$$PI = (-3.410 \times 1.54) + (0.99 \times 1) - (0.038 \times 50) - (0.059 \times 35) + (0.09 \times 20) = -6.4$$

2. Find the probability of survival at 1 year for the patient's score (these data were extrapolated from Figure 2 in the original article).

Score	Approximate probability of 1-year survival
≤ −10	>95%
−10 to −7.5	80–95%
−7.4 to −6	40–80%
> −6	<40%

15

Renal Disease

RENAL LITHIASIS

Ureteral Calculi

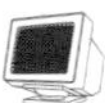

Clinical question

Which patients undergoing intravenous pyelography (IVP) for nontraumatic abdominal or flank pain will have ureteral calculi?

Population and setting

Patients presenting to the emergency department with nontraumatic abdominal or flank pain who underwent an IVP (while the investigator was present) were included. The mean age was 44 years; 69% were male.

Study size

The training group had 203 patients and the validation group 72.

Pretest probability

Altogether, 81% of patients had ureterolithiasis.

Type of validation

Grade II: The validation group was a separate sample from the same population, with data for the validation group gathered prospectively.

Comments

This is a well designed, well validated clinical rule. Note, though, the high pretest probability of stones. Just guessing that everyone had a stone would make you right 81% of the time.

Reference

Elton TJ, Roth CS, Berquist TH, Silverstein MD. A clinical prediction rule for the diagnosis of ureteral calculi in emergency departments. J Gen Intern Med 1993;8:57–62.

CLINICAL PREDICTION RULE

1. Add up the number of points for your patient.

Symptom	Points
Positive KUB (kidneys, uterer, bladder) radiograph	2
Hematuria	2
Flank pain	1
Acute onset	1
Total:	

2. Use the table below to interpret the results.

Score	% With stones
6	98.5
5	96.0
4	90.0

URINARY TRACT INFECTION

Urinary Tract Infection in Women

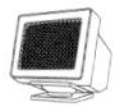

Clinical question

Which women presenting with urinary symptoms have a urinary tract infection (UTI)?

Population and setting

Women over age 14 presenting to the emergency department with suspected UTI were included. The mean age was 27 years (range 14–78 years).

Study size

The training group had 216 patients and the validation group 236.

Pretest probability

Of the validation group, 61% had a UTI, based on the results of a urine culture.

Type of validation

Grade II: The validation group was a separate sample from the same population, with data for the validation group gathered prospectively.

Comments

Most women who think they have a UTI are right. This rule helps us refine our estimates. We can focus on alternative diagnoses such as urethritis or vaginitis if the probability of UTI is low.

Reference

Wigton RS, Hoellerich VL, Omato JP, Leu V, Mazzotta LA, Cheng IH. Use of clinical findings in the diagnosis of urinary tract infection in women. Arch Intern Med 1985;145:2222–2227.

CLINICAL PREDICTION RULE

1. Add up the number of points for your patient.

Symptom	Points
History of UTI	1
Back pain	1
>15 Urinary WBC/HPF	1
>5 Urinary RBC/HPF	1
> A few bacteria in the urine	1
Total:	

WBC = white blood cells; HPF = high-power field.

2. Use the table below to interpret the results.

Score	% With UTI
4–5	86
3	76
2	56
1	25
0	0

END-STAGE RENAL DISEASE

Prognosis for Patients Beginning Dialysis

Clinical question

What is the prognosis for patients with end-stage renal disease (ESRD) beginning renal dialysis?

Population and setting

This Canadian study identified patients from one of eleven centers. They were enrolled when they were diagnosed with ESRD or when they began dialysis (62% hemodialysis, 38% peritoneal dialysis). Of 822 patients, vital status could be determined for 820 at 6 months and 818 at study end; 59% were male; 80% were white; mean age was 58 years.

Study size

Altogether, 822 patients were studied.

Pretest probability

The overall mortality rate at 6 months was 13.7%.

Type of validation

Grade II: The test set was a separate sample from the same population, with data for the test set gathered prospectively.

Comments

The rule was developed from retrospective data and then prospectively validated. It is important to understand that half of all patients with the worst scores were still alive at 6 months, so this rule should not be used to ration care. It does identify patients who require particularly close follow-up.

Reference

Barrett BJ, Parfrey PS, Morgan J, et al. Prediction of early death in end-stage renal disease patients starting dialysis. Am J Kidney Dis 1997;29:214–222.

CLINICAL PREDICTION RULE

1. Calculate your patient's risk score.

Variable	Points
Age (years)	
≤50	1
51–60	2
61–70	3
>70	4
Heart failure	
Heart failure symptoms on strenuous or prolonged activity, or prior heart failure	1
Heart failure on ordinary activity or at rest, or recurrent admissions in heart failure	2
Angina	
New-onset or stable angina or myocardial infarct more than 6 months previously	1
Unstable angina or myocardial infarct less than 6 months previously	2
Treated arrhythmia present	2
Gangrene; inoperable, or surgery for peripheral vascular disease less than 6 months previously	2
Metastatic malignancy, refractory myeloma, or blood dyscrasia	2
Requires mechanical ventilation and/or in coma	4
Severe liver disease and/or in shock	4
Total (range 1–22 points):	

2. The prognosis for patients with this risk score is shown below (percentages are abstracted from a survival curve and may vary by 1–2%).

	% survival at thru time points		
Risk score	50 Days	6 Months	1 Year
0–4	97%	95%	90%
5–9	88%	71%	62%
>9	57%	46%	46%

16

Surgery and Trauma

TRAUMA

Prognosis of Pediatric Head Injury

Clinical question

Which children with head injury will have a good recovery?

Population and setting

Consecutive children with severe head injury and either impairment of consciousness or skull fracture presenting to the major accident unit of a British hospital were included. The mean age was 8.3 years, (range 4 months to 15 years).

Study size

The validation group had 95 patients.

Pretest probability

Of these patients, 11.6% died, and 3.1% had moderate or severe disability.

Type of validation

Grade I: The validation group was from a distinct population. The rule was developed in one group of patients and validated in another.

Comments

This is an implementation of the Glasgow Coma Score, applying it to head-injured children. It includes evaluations at initial presentation and 24 hours later. It is well validated and provides a useful prognostic estimate.

Reference

Grewal M, Sutcliffe AJ. Early prediction of outcome following head injury in children: an assessment of the value of Glasgow Coma Scale score trend and abnormal plantar and pupillary light refleces. J Pediatr Surg 1991;26:1161–1163.

CLINICAL PREDICTION RULE

1. Add up the points in each section for a Glasgow Coma Score (GCS) between 3 and 15. Do this on admission to the hospital and repeat it after 24 hours to assess whether there is any deterioration.

Patient characteristic	Points
Eyes open	
Spontaneously	4
To speech	3
To pain	2
Never	1
Best verbal response	
Oriented	5
Confused	4
Inappropriate words	3
Incomprehensible sounds	2
Silent	1
Best motor response	
Obeys commands	6
Localizes pain	5
Flexion withdrawal	4
Decerebrate flexion	3
Decerebrate extension	2
No response	1
Total:	

2. Find your patient in the following table (numbers shown are the number in each category for each score, total = 95).

GCS score on admission and trend during first 24 hours after injury	Death	Severe disability	Moderate disability	Good recovery
5 or more, with no deterioration	0	1	0	73
5 or more, with deterioration	3	1	0	6
3 or 4	8	0	1	2

Prognosis of Pediatric Near-drowning

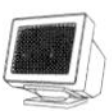

Clinical question

Which children experiencing near-drowning will have a bad outcome (death or vegetative state)?

Population and setting

Consecutive children admitted following submersion in non-icy waters to a tertiary pediatric referral center in Seattle, Washington were included; 72 were comatose on admission. Children dying prior to admission or in the emergency department were excluded. The median age was 2.6 years (range 5 months to 18 years).

Study size

Altogether, 194 patients were studied.

Pretest probability

Among the patients, 27.3% had a bad outcome (death or vegetative state).

Type of validation

Grade IV: The training group was used as the validation group.

Comments

Although this rule is not prospectively validated, it is the only study on this topic and can provide some prognostic information for parents and physicians.

Reference

Graf WD, Cummings P, Quan L, Brutocao D. Predicting outcome in pediatric submersion victims. Ann Emerg Med 1995;26:312–319.

CLINICAL PREDICTION RULE

1. Was the patient comatose on admission? If patients were not comatose on admission, they did not have a bad outcome (death or vegetative state)

2. If comatose on admission, calculate the risk score:
   Pupillary reflex: 0 if present, 1 if absent
   Blood glucose: mg/dl
   Gender: 0 if female, 1 if male

$$\text{Risk score} = 1/\{1 + \exp[6.38 - (4.23 \times \text{pupil reflex}) - (0.01 \times \text{blood glucose}) - (2.3 \times \text{gender})]\}$$

3. A range of risk scores are calculated below:

		Score, by blood glucose on admission (mg/dl)							
Pupillary reflex	Gender	100	150	200	250	300	400	500	600
Present	Male	0.04	0.07	0.11	0.17	0.25	0.48	0.72	0.87
Absent	Male	0.76	0.84	0.90	0.93	**0.96**	**0.98**	**0.99**	**1.00**
Present	Female	0.00	0.01	0.01	0.02	0.03	0.08	0.20	0.41
Absent	Female	0.24	0.34	0.46	0.59	0.70	0.86	**0.95**	**0.98**

The numbers in boldface represent a risk score: ≥0.95.

4. Interpret the score using the following table for comatose patients.

Risk score	Bad outcome (death or vegetative state)	Favorable outcome (all other outcomes)
≥0.95	93 (48%)	0
<0.95	50 (26%)	50 (26%)

The rule is 65% sensitive and 100% specific for prediction of bad outcome. It is more useful when positive (≥0.95).

Predicting Seat Belt Usage

Clinical question

Which patients do not wear seat belts and would benefit from directed patient education?

Population and setting

Adults in Tennessee completing a voluntary health risk appraisal (mostly state employees) were included. Only 11% were African American.

Study size

The training group had 1554 patients and the validation group 1554.

Pretest probability

Altogether, 33% reported low seat-belt use (less than 25% utilization).

Type of validation

Grade III: The validation group was a separate sample from the same population, although data for both training and validation groups were gathered at the same time.

Comments

This is an interesting rule because of the topic: predicting a behavior such as seat belt use. It could conceivably be implemented as part of an initial outpatient assessment to identify patients who should receive counseling about seat belt use.

Reference

Lichtenstein MJ, Bolton A, Wade G. Derivation and validation of a clinical prediction rule for predicting seat belt utilization. J Fam Pract 1989;28:289–292.

CLINICAL PREDICTION RULE

1. Multiply the cofactor in column A by the coefficient in column B and put the result in the "subtotal" column.

Question	Column A		Column B	Subtotal
Age at last birthday (years)?	No. of years		0.24	
How often do you use drugs or medications that affect your mood or help you to relax?	Almost every day =	1	4.09	
	Sometimes =	2		
	Rarely or never =	3		
Miles per year as a driver and/or passenger (10,000 = average)	0–10,000 =	1	5.08	
	10,001–20,000 =	2		
	>20,000 =	3		
Education: schooling completed	Grade school only =	1	11.18	
	Completed high school =	2		
	Some college =	3		
	College or professional degree =	4		
Race/origin	White (non-Hispanic) =	1	−18.31	
	Black =	2		
Tobacco use: average no. of cigarettes smoked per day during the last 5 years (ex-smokers should use the last 5 years before quitting)	None =	0	−2.73	
	1–10 =	1		
	11–20 =	2		
	>21 =	3		
In general, how satisfied are you with your life?	Mostly satisfied =	1	−3.50	
	Partly satisfied =	2		
	Mostly disappointed =	3		
	Not sure =	4		
Body mass index	Weight (kg)/height^2 (m^2)		−0.83	
Urban or rural residence	Urban =	1	−4.08	
	Rural =	2		
			Total:	

2. Find the score in the table (shown are numbers with a given score in each utilization group, and the likelihood ratio (LR) for being in the low utilization group in the final column; high LR means lower likelihood of seat belt use):

	Seat belt use (no. of subjects)			
Score	0–25% Utilization	26–75% Utilization	76–100% Utilization	LR for 0–25% Utilization
≤−1	57	83	146	3.31
0–9	100	95	128	1.65
10–18	123	89	93	0.98
19–25	170	77	77	0.59
>26	196	63	57	0.38

Likelihood of Major Trauma

Clinical question

Which injured patients are at risk for death or the need for emergent operation?

Population and setting

Training group: consecutive adults (age > 14 years) admitted to a university trauma center by land ambulance system; mean age 31 years; 42% were female.

Validation set: 1275 trauma patients over age 15 were studied at an urban medical center (MetroHealth in Cleveland), but sufficient data to calculate the score were available for only 1027; 659 were male, 368 female; average age 34.4 years.

Study size

A total of 1004 patients were used to develop the rule. The validation study by Emerman et al. used 1027 patients.

Pretest probability

The risk of death in the validation study was 37/1027 (3.6%), and the number needing emergent operation was 38/1027 (3.7%); 46/1027 (4.5%) either died or required emergent operation.

Type of validation

Grade I: The validation group was from a distinct population. The rule was developed in one group of patients and validated in another.

Comments

Although the original study of Baxt et al. lacks prospective validation, the later validation study by Emerman et al. provides that, and shows that the rule remains accurate and useful.

References

Baxt WG, Jones G, Fortlage D. The Trauma Triage Rule: a new, resource-based approach to the prehospital identification of major trauma victims. Ann Emerg Med 1990;19:1401–1406.

Emerman C, Shade B, Kubincanek J. Comparative performance of the Baxt Trauma Triage Rule. Am J Emerg Med 1992;10:294–297.

CLINICAL PREDICTION RULE

1. The Baxt Trauma Triage Rule is positive if in the prehospital setting the patient has
   Systolic blood pressure < 85 mm Hg *or*
   Glasgow Coma Score, motor subscore, < 5 *or*
   Potential penetrating injury of the head, neck, or trunk

2. Use the following table to interpret the rule.

		Dying or requiring emergent operation	
Trauma triage rule	Likelihood ratio	Overall rate of death/ emergent operation = 4.5%	Overall rate of death/ emergent operation = 2.3%
Positive	8.5	28.5%	16.6%
Negative	0.07	0.4%	0.2%

If the overall rate of death or emergent operation among adult trauma patients is 4.5% at your institution, the percent of patients with a positive Trauma Triage Rule who will die or require emergent surgery is 28.5%.

Prehospital Index for Trauma

Clinical question

Which injured patients are at risk for death or the need for emergent operation?

Population and setting

A series of 1275 trauma patients over age 15 were studied at an urban medical center (MetroHealth in Cleveland), but sufficient data to calculate the score were available for only 1027; 659 were male, 368 female; average age was 34.4 years.

Study size

The validation set had 1027 patients.

Pretest probability

The risk of death in the validation study was 37/1027 (3.6%), and the number needing emergent operation was 38/1027 (3.7%); 46/1027 (4.5%) either died or required emergent operation.

Type of validation

Grade I: The validation group was from a distinct population. The rule was developed in one group of patients and validated in another.

Comments

This is a prospective validation of a clinical rule for prehospital triage of trauma patients. It is similar to the Baxt Trauma Triage Rule in accuracy but is somewhat more complicated.

References

Emerman C, Shade B, Kubincanek J. Comparative performance of the Baxt Trauma Triage Rule. Am J Emerg Med 1992;10:294–297.

Koehler JJ, Baer L, Malafa S, et al. Prehospital index: a scoring system for field triage of trauma victims. Ann Emerg Med 1986;15:178–182.

CLINICAL PREDICTION RULE

1. Calculate the patient's Prehospital Index Score (range 0–24 points).

Variable	Points
Systolic blood pressure (mm Hg)	
>100	0
86–100	1
75–85	2
0–74	5
Pulse (beats/min)	
51–119	0
>120	3
<50	5
Consciousness	
Normal	0
Confused/combative	3
No intelligible words	5
Penetrating chest/abdominal injury	
Yes	4
No	0
Total:	

2. Use the following table to interpret the rule.

		Dying or requiring emergent operation	
Prehospital index	Likelihood ratio	Overall rate of death/ emergent operation = 4.5%	Overall rate of death/ emergent operation = 2.3%
>3	7.8	26.7%	15.4%
0–2	0.07	0.4%	0.2%

If the overall rate of death or emergent operation among adult trauma patients is 4.5% at your institution, the percent of patients with a prehospital index > 3 who will die or require emergent surgery is 26.7%.

Example: A patient with systolic blood pressure 120 mm Hg, pulse 130 beats/min, confusion and combativeness but no penetrating injury would get 0 + 3 + 3 + 0 = 6 points and have a "positive" score (>3).

Prognosis after Major Trauma

Clinical question

Which patients admitted for major trauma will be alive at 21 days?

Population and setting

Patients who had been examined neurologically and assessed for the Innsbruck Coma Score following major trauma were included. They were excluded if hypothermic (core temperature < 34°C), in severe shock (systolic blood pressure < 80 mm Hg), or had received sedatives prior to the examination. The mean age was 33.5 years (range 1–87 years); 71% were male.

Study size

The validation group had 421 patients.

Pretest probability

The overall mortality rate was 46.8%.

Type of validation

Grade I: The validation group was from a distinct population. The rule was developed in one group of patients and validated in another.

Comments

This rule was well validated on a large group of patients.

Reference

Benzer A, Mitterschiffthaler G, Marosi M, et al. Prediction of non-survival after trauma: Innsbruck Coma Scale. Lancet 1991;338:977–978.

CLINICAL PREDICTION RULE

1. Calculate the Innsbruck Coma Score for your patient (oral automatisms are not included in this version of the score because only patients in a nonvegetative state are included).

Neurologic assessment	Score
Reaction to acoustic stimuli	
Turning toward stimuli	3
Better-than-extension movements	2
Extension movements	1
None	0
Reaction to pain	
Defensive movements	3
Better-than-extension movements	2
Extension movements	1
None	0
Body posture	
Normal	3
Better-than-extension movements	2
Extension movements	1
Flaccid	0
Eye opening	
Spontaneous	3
To acoustic stimuli	2
To pain stimuli	1
None	0
Pupil size	
Normal	3
Narrow	2
Dilated	1
Completely dilated	0
Pupil response to light	
Sufficient	3
Reduced	2
Minimum	1
No response	0
Position and movements of eyeballs	
Fixing with eyes	3
Sway of eyeballs	2
Divergent	1
Divergent fixed	0
Total ICS score:	

2. Outcomes for each range of ICS score is shown below.

ICS score	No. surviving/total
0–1	0/79 (0%)
2–3	5/38 (13%)
4–5	8/32 (25%)
≥6	211/272 (78%)

■ POSTOPERATIVE INFECTION AND PERITONITIS

Bacterial Infection after Abdominal Surgery

Clinical question

Which febrile patients who have had abdominal surgery have a bacterial infection?

Population and setting

A random selection of adult patients who underwent abdominal surgery at a university medical center were included. Patients were excluded if they underwent pelvic or gynecologic surgery. Of the 434 patients, 25% were under age 40, 52% were age 40–70 years, and 23% were over age 70; 54% were male.

Study size

A series of 434 patients were studied, of whom 163 developed postoperative fever.

Pretest probability

Of the patients with postoperative fever, 16% had a bacterial infection.

Type of validation

Grade IV: The training group was used as the validation group.

Comments

This study is limited by the lack of validation, and it should be used with caution.

Reference

Mellors JW, Kelly JJ, Gusberg RJ, Horwitz SM, Horwitz RI. A simple index to estimate the likelihood of bacterial infection in patients developing fever after abdominal surgery. Am Surg 1988;54:558–564.

CLINICAL PREDICTION RULE

1. Count the number of features your patient has.

Variable	Points
WBC < 5000 or > 10,000/mm^3	1
Postop increase in BUN > 25%	1
Postop BUN > mg/dl	1
Trauma	1
Fever onset after second postop day	1
American Society of Anesthesiologists (ASA) preoperative physical status class III–V[a]	1
Initial fever ≥ 38.6°C	1
Total:	

WBC = which blood cell count; BUN = blood urea nitrogen.
[a]American Society of Anesthesiologists. New classification of physical status. Anesthesiology 1963;24:111.

2. The likelihood that fever represents bacterial infection is as follows.

Points	Patients with infection
0	1/50 (2%)
1	12/88 (14%)
2	10/22 (45%)
3	3/3 (100%)

Peritonitis

Clinical question

Which patients with peritonitis are at high risk for death and may require more aggressive intervention?

Population and setting

Patients with peritonitis at one of seven surgical centers in three European countries for whom complete data were available were included.

Study size

The validation group included 2003 patients.

Pretest probability

There was a 19.5% overall mortality rate.

Type of validation

Grade I: The validation group was from a distinct population. The rule was developed in one group of patients and validated in another.

Comments

There is some potential for misinterpretation of some of the predictor variables (origin of sepsis, diffuse generalized peritonitis, exudate characteristics). Otherwise this is a well validated clinical rule.

References

Billing A, Frohlich D, Schildberg FW, Peritonitis Study Group. Prediction of outcome using the Mannheim peritonitis index in 2003 patients. Br J Surg 1994;81:209–213.

Bosscha K, Reijders K, Hulstaert F, Algra A, van der Werken C. Prognosic scoring systems to predict outcome in peritonitis and intra-abdominal sepsis. Br J Surg 1997;84:1532–1534.

CLINICAL PREDICTION RULE

1. Add up the points below for your patient.

Risk factor	Points
Age > 50 years	5
Female gender	5
Organ failure[a]	7
Malignancy	4
Preoperative duration of peritonitis > 24 hours	4
Origin of sepsis not colonic	4
Diffuse generalized peritonitis	6
Exudate (choose one only)	
Clear	0
Cloudy, purulent	6
Fecal	12
Total:	

[a]Definition of organ failure:
Kidney: serum creatinine ≥ 177 μmol/L (1.5 mg/dl) or urine output <20 ml/hr
Lung: PO_2 < 50 mm Hg or PCO_2 > 50 mm Hg
Shock: hypodynamic or hyperdynamic
Intestinal obstruction (only if profound): paralysis ≥ 24 hours or complete mechanical ileus

2. Find the mortality corresponding to your patient's score.

Mannheim peritonitis Index	No. of patients	Mortality
<21	966	2.3%
21–29	664	22.5%
>29	373	59.1%

A subsequent independent validation of 50 patients in a Dutch hospital found the following outcome.

Mannheim peritonitis Index	Deaths/total with that score
0–26	1/15 (6.7%)
≥27	21/35 (60.0%)

Deciding to Reoperate: Abdominal Reoperation Predictive Index

Clinical question

When does a critically ill patient require reoperation following major abdominal surgery?

Population and setting

Consecutive critically ill patients admitted after major abdominal surgery over a span of 5 years to the intensive care unit (ICU) of a teaching hospital in Buenos Aires were studied. The mean age was 64 years; approximately 61% were female. The most common findings at the primary operation were peritonitis (30%), biliary obstruction (15%), intestinal obstruction (14%), gastrointestinal tract cancer (11%), urologic disease (7%), and esophagogastroduodenal disease (7%).

Study size

A series of 542 patients were studied to determine the value of the clinical rule and algorithm.

Pretest probability

In the original validation, 38% of patients required reoperation.

Type of validation

Grade IV: The training group was used as the validation group.

Comments

The authors developed a predictive index in a previous study. In this one they compare an algorithm based on it to usual care. They found reduced mortality (35% vs. 45%) and reduced length of stay in the ICU among those managed using the algorithm. However, the control used was a historical one: Patients from 1984 and 1985 were the controls, and those from 1985 to 1989 were the experimental group. This rule has considerable promise but should be prospectively validated before application at your institution.

Reference

Pusajo JF, Bumaschny E, Doglio GR, et al. Postoperative intra-abdominal sepsis requiring reoperation: value of a predictive index. Arch Surg 1993;128:218–222.

CLINICAL PREDICTION RULE

1. Determine your patient's Abdominal Reoperation Predictive Index (ARPI).

Variable	Points
Emergency surgery (at primary operation)	3
Respiratory failure	2
Renal failure	2
Ileus (from 72 hours after surgery)	4
Abdominal pain (from 48 hours after surgery)	5
Wound infection	8
Consciousness alterations	2
Symptoms appearing from the 4th day after surgery	6
ARPI score:	

2. The following algorithm was used to guide the management of patients immediately after major abdominal surgery presenting sudden or progressive deterioration in their general condition ("special studies" include laboratory assays and imaging studies).

ARPI score	Management strategy
1–10	Patients were observed. If symptoms persisted, special studies were ordered. If positive, reoperate; if negative, continue observation.
11–15	Special studies were performed. If positive, reoperate, if negative, observe; if symptoms persist, reoperate.
16–20	Special studies were performed, followed by reoperation.
>20	Reoperation.

Appendix A

Using RuleRetriever Software

One way to make clinical prediction rules more useful is to put them on a computer. Simply checking off a few boxes and pressing a button gives us a clinical prediction, and there is no need to memorize rules or carry them with us. This book is accompanied by software for the Windows 95/98/NT operating systems that implements many of the most useful clinical prediction rules from this book. Although the software is not needed to use the clinical prediction rules in this book, it is a useful complement, particularly for rules that involve complex calculations.

■ IMPORTANT NOTE

Because information is on a computer does not make it right. When using the results of a clinical prediction rule, whether from the book itself or the software, remember that it is only one piece of information. You must use it in the context of all other information about the patient and with your best clinical judgment. The rules are not guaranteed to be correct all the time (or even any of the time).

Installing RuleRetriever for Windows 95/98/NT

To install the software for the Windows 95/98/NT operating system, put the enclosed CD-ROM disk in your computer. There are two ways to do it.

Method 1

1. From the Start Menu, select Settings, Control Panel.
2. Double-click on the Add/Remove programs icon.
3. Type in D:\RuleSetup.exe, where d: is the letter of your CD-ROM drive.

Method 2

1. Select Run from the Start Menu
2. Type in D:\RuleSetup.exe, where d: is the letter of your CD-ROM drive.

Follow the simple instructions in each setup program, and the software will be installed on your hard drive in the Program Files\RuleRetriever\ folder.

Running RuleRetriever for Windows 95/98/NT

To run RuleRetriever, select Programs from the Start Menu, then select RuleRetriever, then RuleRetriever. You will see the opening screen:

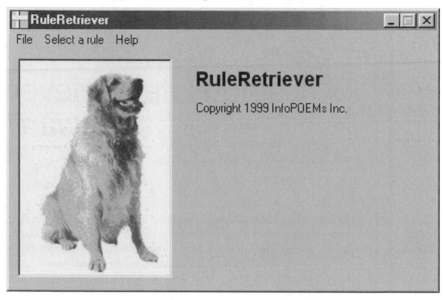

To exit the program, press the "x" in the upper right corner or select "Exit" from the File menu. To minimize the program, press the minimize icon in the upper right corner of the dialog box.

To select a rule, click on "Select a rule." For a simple example, select Infectious diseases. You will see a second menu open with two items; select "Diagnosis of strep throat." When you select this item, you will see the following screen.

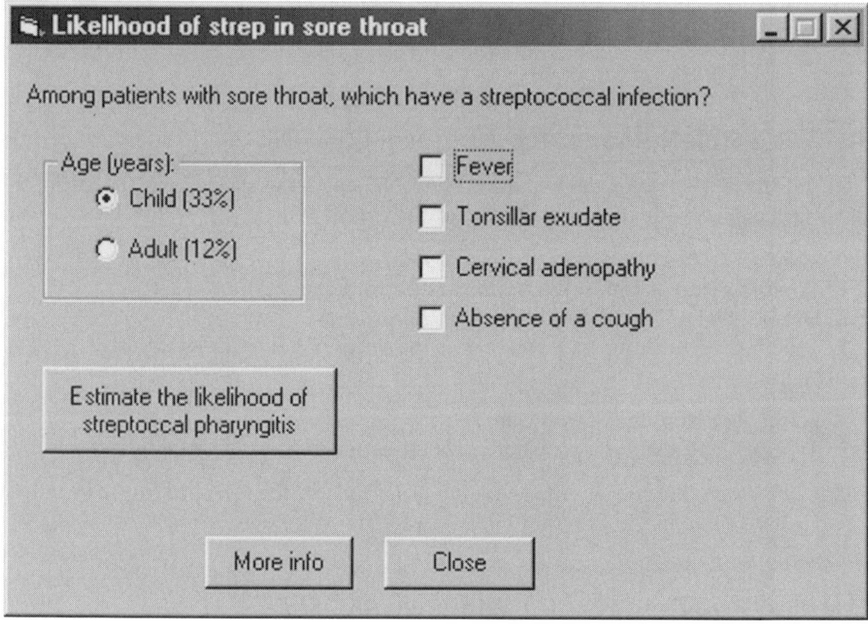

Let us say we have an adult patient with fever and cough but no tonsillar exudate or cervical adenopathy. You would select "Adult" and then check the "Fever" box. Note that the fourth checkbox is "*Absence* of cough," so you would not check it (our patient is coughing). The screen will now look like this.

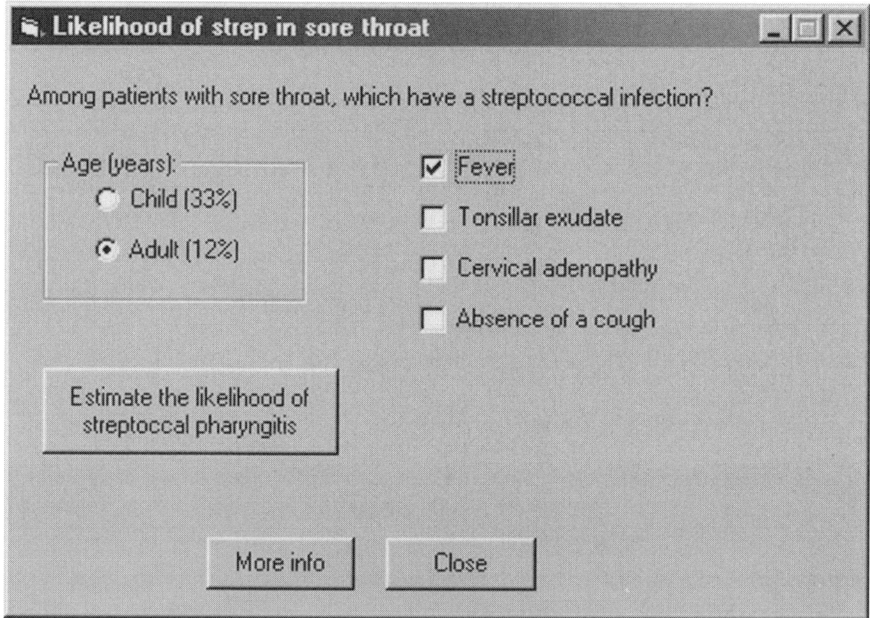

Pressing the button labeled "Estimate the likelihood of streptococcal pharyngitis" will give you an estimate.

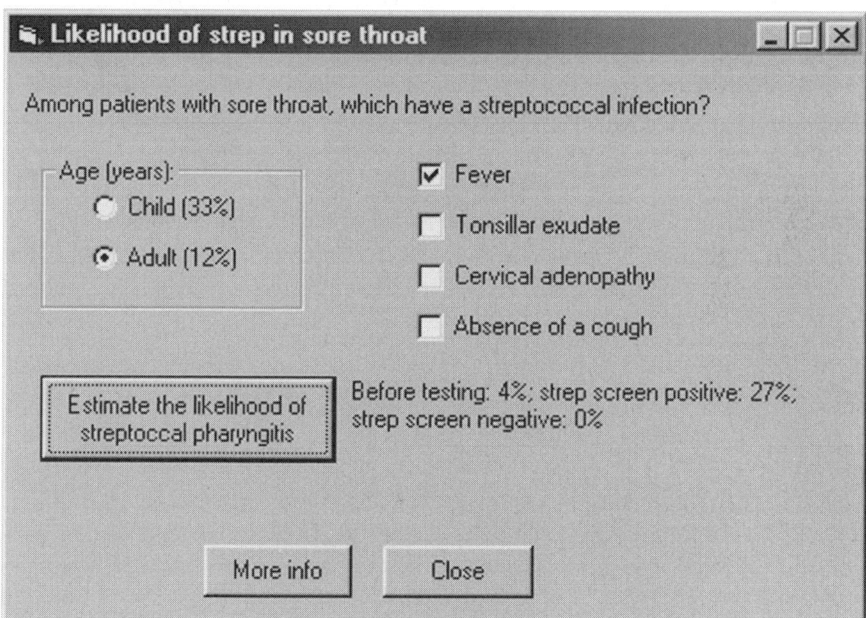

The calculator gives you the probability of strep based on the clinical examination alone (4%) and the probability, given a positive or negative strep screen. The strep screen calculations assume a sensitivity and specificity of 90%.

Do you want to know more about how this rule was developed and validated? Just press the "More info" button:

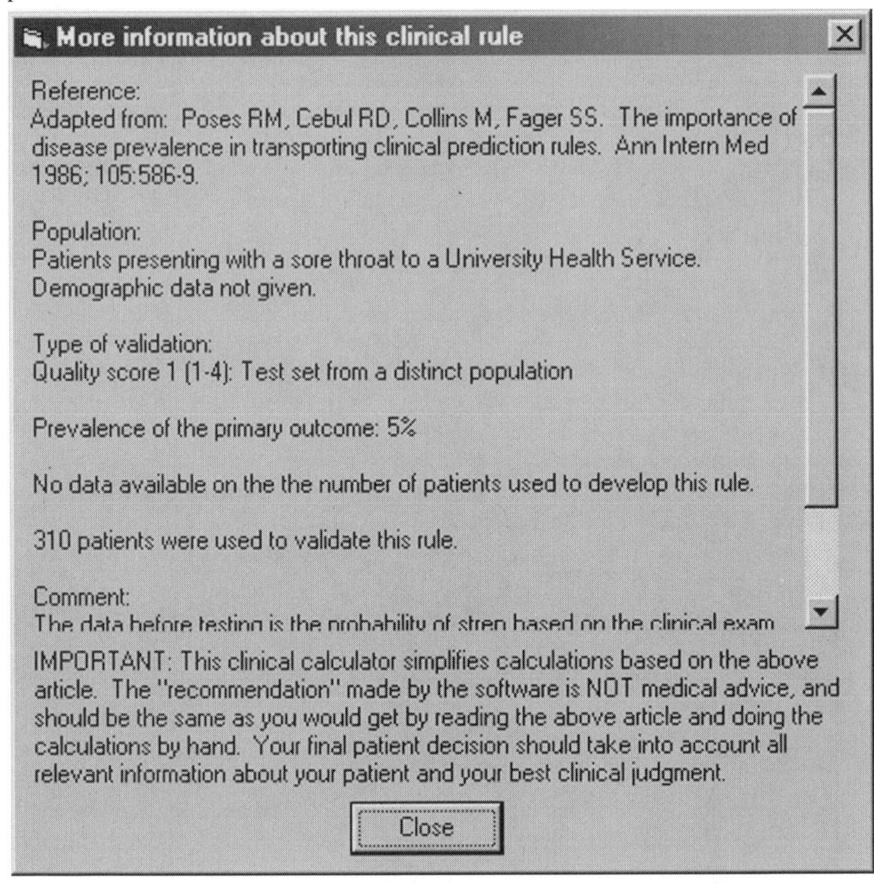

Let us look at a more complex clinical rule. Close the "Strep" and "More Info" windows by selecting "Close" for each. You should now see the main window again:

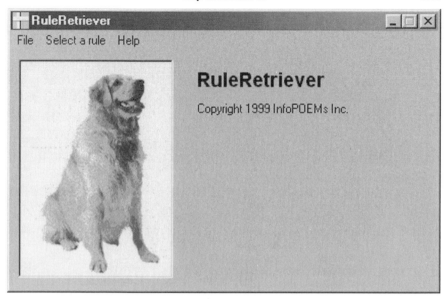

Open the "Select a rule menu," and then select "Cardiovascular diseases." Next, select "Coronary artery disease," followed by "Risk of CAD, MI, and CHF (Framingham data)" from the submenu. You will see the following window:

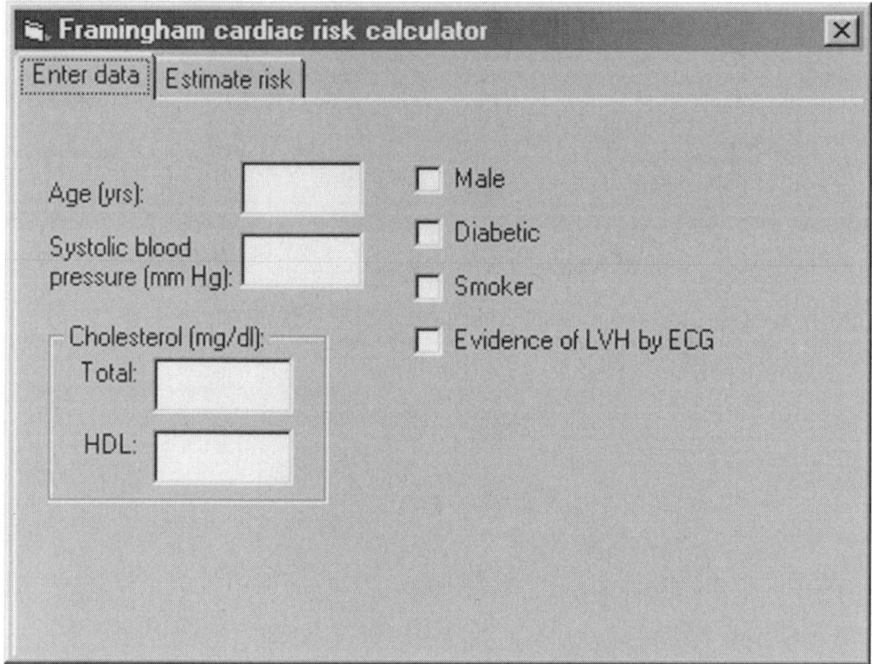

If your patient is a 38-year-old male nonsmoker with a systolic blood pressure of 135 mm Hg, total cholesterol of 220 mg/dl, and HDL-cholesterol of 45 mg/dl, you should fill in the screen to look like this.

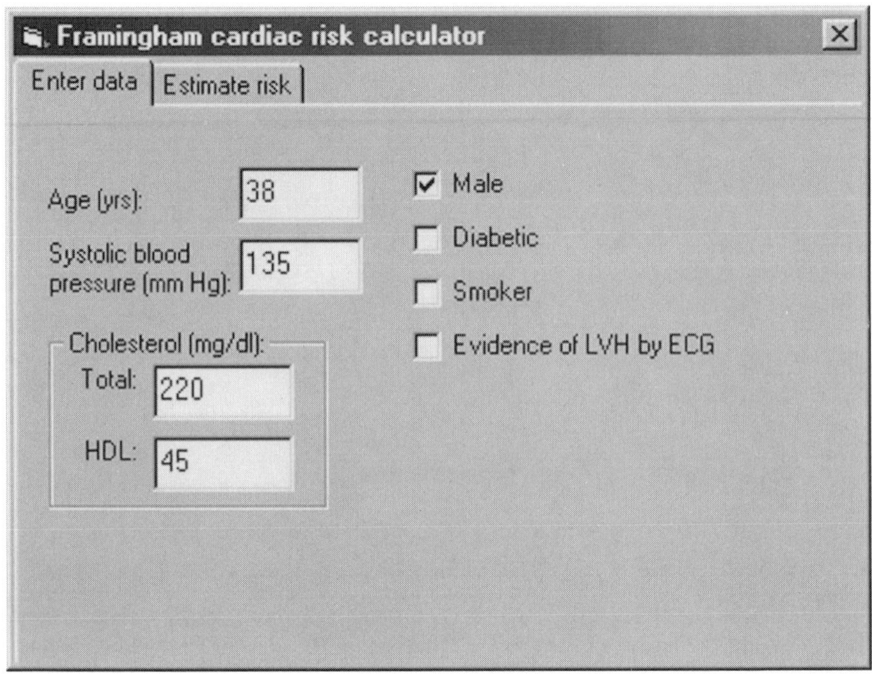

Next, click on "Estimate risk" tab. This tabbed view allows us to fit more information in a small area and works much like the tabbed folders in your file drawer. After clicking on "Estimate risk" click on "Estimate 10 year risk."

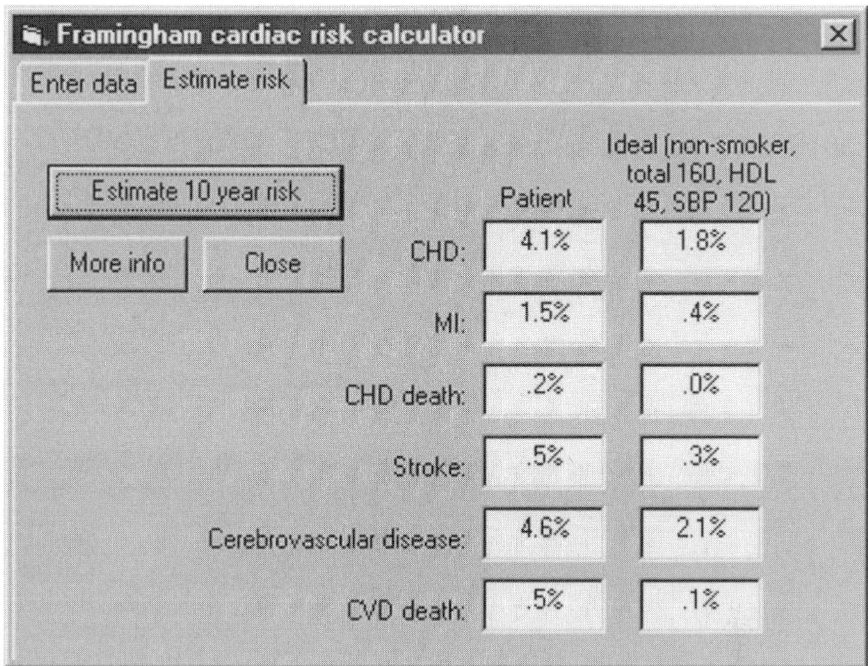

The above window gives you an estimate of the probability of each of the events (coronary heart disease, myocardial infarction, and so on) occurring during the next 10 years. The risk of these events for an optimal risk profile (same age and gender as the patient, but nonsmoker, normal blood pressure, and excellent lipid profile) is shown for comparison.

Appendix B

InfoRetriever Demo

The CD-ROM that accompanies this book includes a demonstration version of InfoRetriever for Windows 95/98/NT. In addition to the clinical rules featured in the InfoRetriever Special Edition software, it also includes:

- More than 1000 synopses of the recent primary care literature from Evidence-Based Practice
- More than 700 abstracts from the Cochrane Database of Systematic Reviews
- Basic prescribing information for more than 1200 drugs
- A handy diagnostic test calculator
- Selected summaries of evidence-based clinical prediction rules
- Collected POEMs critical appraisals from the *Journal of Family Practice*

You can use the demo software 10 times. To learn how to subscribe to InfoRetriever, and to download the latest version, go to the InfoRetriever Web site at http://www.infopoems.com. It costs only $149 and includes a full year of free updates to keep your information up-to-date. To install InfoRetriever:

1. Select Run from the Start Menu.
2. Type d:\Irsetup.exe, where d is the letter of your CD-ROM drive.
3. Follow the installation instructions. You may have to reboot your computer and rerun the installation if certain files are in use.

Index